True Stories Of A Small-Town Veterinarian

MENDING
GOD'S CREATURES

James A. Roloff, DVM

YorkshirePublishing
www.yorkshirepublishing.com
Write Now.

For permission requests, write to the publisher at the address below.

Yorkshire Publishing
3207 South Norwood Avenue
Tulsa, Oklahoma 74135
www.YorkshirePublishing.com
918.394.2665

CONTENTS

DEDICATION

This book is dedicated to my lovely wife, Sandy. It was her faithful support, encouragement, willing sacrifices, and sincere compassion for animals that inspired and sustained me through the years. Together we achieved our hopes and dreams.

ACKNOWLEDGEMENTS

A special thank you goes to all the receptionists, veterinary assistants, veterinary technicians, and veterinarians for their conscientious efforts and professionalism throughout the years. I couldn't have done it without you, and I'm eternally grateful for your devoted service.

Veterinary Technicians, Veterinary Assistants, and Receptionists

Angela, Barb, Chandra, Christine, Darlene, Donna S., Donna SL., Heather S., Heather W., Heidi, Hillary, Ivy, Janice, Jennifer, Kathleen, Megan, Melanie, Melody, Merle, Rachel M., Rachael Mc., Robbie, Sarah, Sharon, Tami, Taryn, Tauni, Vashon, Vickie, Whitney, and Candace, our special friend and consultant.

Associate Veterinarians

Dr. Al, Dr. Bill ("Wild Bill"), Dr. Dee, Dr. Kate, Dr. Paul

PREFACE

What defines a true friend? To many of us, our animal companions are true friends because they often demonstrate that supreme measure of devotion, – unconditional love. They can give us joy, provide us with peace and comfort, and teach us how to be more forgiving. In many cases, they inspire us to be better individuals. Many years ago, Chief Seattle of the Suquamesh Indian Tribe said it perfectly:

"What is man without the beasts?
If all the beasts were gone, men would die from
great loneliness of spirit.
For whatever happens to the beasts will soon
happen to man.
All things are connected."

Growing up on a farm provided me an opportunity to interact with all kinds of animals. It wasn't long before I sensed a definite connection with them. They were my friends, and witnessing them battle pain, sickness, and disease inspired me to find a way to relieve the discomfort and provide healing, hence the calling to become a veterinarian.

THE LETTER

"Time stands still for no man." I forget who actually said that, but it is certainly true. That burning desire, down deep inside, to become a veterinarian was never quenched. I was twenty-six years old, married to a beautiful young lady, had a young son, and had recently graduated from Eastern Washington University, having completed a four-year premed curriculum with a major in Biology. I'd applied to the Washington State University College of Veterinary Medicine, gone through the admissions interviews, and was at the mercy of the selection board. It was a well-known fact that many students weren't accepted on their first application, but I was still hopeful, although somewhat apprehensive.

This whole thing of striving for that goal of becoming a veterinarian had been a major sacrifice for all of us, – Sandy, Eric, and myself. We had been through four years of doing without a lot of things, and now, if I got accepted into vet school, we'd have four more lean years to endure. We were willing. We were a team. Even though we were poor financially and drove a clunker, we were rich in hope and faith. Now, all we had to do was wait patiently for that letter. It was difficult going to the mailbox daily and finding it empty. Would I be one of the lucky ones to get accepted on my first application, or would I have to find a farm job and reapply the following year? Could I ask Sandy and Eric to hang on for another year while many other guys my age were now gainfully employed? Those were very sobering questions that kept running through my mind.

Then one beautiful day, as I opened the mailbox, – there it was! The letter from Washington State University College of Veterinary Medicine, and it was addressed to me. As I held that envelope in my hands, all the hopes, dreams, and sacrifices of the past, just to get to this point, flashed before my eyes. The first words I saw when I opened the letter were, – "Congratulations, you've been accepted into the College of Veterinary Medicine." I didn't have time to read any further. Tears of joy and relief welled up in my eyes as I showed the letter to Sandy. We made it! Thank you, Lord. As reality sank in, I knew that being accepted into vet school was a major turning point in our lives, and the beginning of a new adventure.

THE COLLEGE DAYS

Veterinary School

The four years of vet school were far from being a cake walk. The introduction speech by one of the vet school profs to our incoming class of sixty students was short, sweet, and definitely to the point. "Do not fall behind! If you do, you'll never catch up!" Believe me, truer words were never spoken. The courses were intense, the professors demanding, and the competition was fierce. There was no let-up for the four years of study. The very high stress level had an adverse effect on some of my classmates, and it unfortunately resulted in them withdrawing from school. The great majority of us, however, endured with determined and committed resolve. The driving forces that kept me going were my love and respect for animals, a good sense of humor, the support and encouragement of my family, and most importantly, my strong faith.

"Red"

It was the anesthesiology laboratory class during my second year of vet school that I first ventured outside the box, and it wouldn't be the last time either! The students were paired up and assigned a dog for the hands-on lab sessions. We were to observe and record the patient's physiological responses to various forms of anesthesia. At the end of the course, these dogs were to be humanely euthanized, because they were essentially owned by the State of Washington, — as we were emphatically told. I had been assigned a young, happy, very energetic Irish Setter, who I later named "Red". He was a real kick in the pants! He loved the attention, and was always excited about going to the laboratory. He'd pull hard on the leash, seemingly looking forward to his next "hit" of anesthesia. I guess you could say that Red had become an anesthesia junkie. I really did like that goofy guy. He was a very good patient, and we sorta connected. The last day of the course had arrived, and it was now time to relinquish the dogs to their un-fortunate fate. As I held Red"s head in my hands and looked into his big brown eyes, I paused momentarily, then told him, "Red, let's get you outta here!" So, I quickly grabbed a leash, and jetted out the door with Red gleefully prancing in tow. He was his usual happy-go-lucky self, looking up at me as if saying, "Oh boy,— Where we goin?" We made it out of the building, — undetected, —and by some act of providence, standing right next to the exit door was a fellow student taking a smoke break. I handed him the leash and said, "Here, take this dog for a short walk for me. OK! Take him somewhere, right now, where I can't see him. I'll catch up with you later and get the dog,— but just get him out of here!" The other student could tell something was up, but thankfully he didn't ask any questions. He just took off with Red, happily pull-ing on the leash, — "Oh boy, I'm goin for a walk". I then went back to the lab to pick up my books, and suddenly encountered the instructor,— standing by the door. "Roloff, where's your dog? You're aware that these dogs are State property, aren't you? If you have that dog, that would be considered stealing from the State of Washington, and you'd be breaking the law" I swallowed hard, — looked the professor straight in the eyes and replied, — "I got rid of him, and I don't know where he is." That was the truth! I didn't know EXACTLY where he was, — at that EXACT moment. So, in my mind, I wasn't lying. Instead, I considered it to be a mat-ter of symantics. The prof just stood there, looking me eyeball to eyeball. The stare-down probably lasted only a few seconds, but it seemed like an eternity to me. I kept telling myself, "Don't sweat! — Don't blink! Finally the prof looked away, shook his head, and I heard him mutter under his breath as he turned to walk away, "Don't get caught." — I didn't, and eventually we found Red a nice home in the country where he could run free and live a carefree life. I'd helped save a friend's life, and I felt good about that, —— and still do.

A Good Laugh!

I'll never forget one particularly humorous incident that occurred during my third year of veterinary school. Jake Burns and I were classmates, and were scheduled to work together on large animal reception one Saturday morning in late September. Our duties were to get the medical histories of the patients, and perform the initial examinations. If any treatments were necessary, we'd do those under the direct supervision of an instructor. Jake and I were hoping for a light caseload that morning, because there was a football game scheduled at Martin Stadium at 2:00 PM, and both of us were planning to go see it. Everything had been going along smoothly up until 11:00 AM.—— Then it happened! An old cattle truck pulled up to the unloading dock, and the stench of rotting afterbirth permeated the air. The cow was unloaded, and placed in the treatment stanchion. The smell was so foul that we had to place menthol rub up our noses to keep from gagging. Naturally, the instructor turned to Jake and I and said, "Boys, now's the time to see what you're made of." Jake gave me a quick glance and rolled his eyes. We both knew what was coming.

The cow's rectal temperature was understandably elevated since she'd become septic from the retained, putrefying, afterbirth tissue. It had to be manually removed, and believe me, that was one messy, stinky job. Jake and I both worked at it, and finally we got all that rotten stuff out of there. The cow was good to go,

5

but we weren't! We stunk to high heaven, even though we wore coveralls and shoulder length obstetric gloves. We didn't notice it at the time, but our coveralls had shrunk somewhat from being washed so much, and now the bottoms of our jeans were exposed, to anything and everything.

We finished up a little late, but still had time to make a quick run home, clean up, and get it to the game on time. I got to the game, and noticed Jake sitting with a group of people in the end zone section. He seemed to be enjoying himself, but as time passed, most of the people around Jake had left. He looked pretty lonely over there, sitting all by himself, so I ventured over to sit with him. When sitting down next to Jake, I got a whiff of that rotten afterbirth stench. So I asked him, "Jake, did you go back to your dorm and clean up, because you smell just like that dang cow?" Jake told me he'd cleaned up, — but as I looked down at the cuffs of his jeans,— there it was. A piece of rotten afterbirth, — stuck on his pantleg. No wonder the people around him took off! They couldn't stand the smell. Jake told me that his sense of smell had never been very good, — No Kidding!!! He tore out a page from his game program, — wiped off his pants, and we had a good laugh. There we were, watching the rest of the game all by ourselves, undisturbed in our own little section, just like two guys in church, sitting in our own pew.

"Rufus", The Elevator Cat

It was the summer between my sophomore and junior years of vet school that I found myself in dire need of earning some extra income. Working while attending vet school was discouraged, so Sandy was our main source of income. She worked as a nurse for a local physician, and had a definite gift of compassion for the patients. I was so proud of her. I applied for summer employment at the Whitman County Grain Growers, hoping that my experiences

6

on a wheat and cattle ranch would help me get hired. It did! The early part of the summer job consisted of getting the elevators prepared for the upcoming harvest season. There were bins to be cleaned, augers repaired, conveyer belts replaced, and holdover grain needed to be loaded into rail cars and shipped out. The hours were long and the labor was intense. My immediate foreman was about eight years younger than myself, had completed only high school, and seemed to delight in calling me, "college boy". Hey, I didn't mind. I respected his position, and I worked hard for him. The company manager noticed my work ethic and placed me in charge of the Fallon elevator during the harvest season. Once again, hard work is noticed, and will be rewarded. On one routine day at the elevator, while sitting in the shade having lunch, I noticed some fast, staccato type movement out of the corner of my eye. My first thought was, —— RAT! I grabbed a nearby shovel, ready for action. Unexpectedly, the head of a young cat peered around the corner. With ears up, eyes opened wide, he bounded towards me from behind his cover, and unabashedly invited himself to share my lunch. So, now I had company for dining. We ate and talked. — I did most of the talking, of course. This little grey shorthair tabby, about four months old, ended up eating most of my food, but I enjoyed our time together. After chowing down as much as possible, he delightedly excused himself and left. The next day, at about the same time, he magically reappeared for more lunch, pets, and conversation. That scenario continued throughout the duration of the harvest season. When the harvest had come to a close, it was time to shut down the elevator, lock up, and go home. As I was getting into my car and about to leave the elevator for the last time, that little lunch buddy suddenly appeared and sauntered toward the car. I'd grown fond of that little moocher, so I held the car door open and asked him, "You comin or stayin?". He jumped right in without a moments hesitation, plopped himself down on the seat, right next to me, as if he'd done it a hundred times before, —— and home we went. We named him "Rufus", and we were the best of friends for many years. Rufus was more of a purr-son than he was a cat, and together we forged wonderful memories that will last forever.

"Rufus", all grown up.

The Gentle Giant

C linical rotations were a part of the veterinary curriculum wherein the third and fourth year veterinary students assisted in the examinations, diagnosis, and treatments of hospitalized cases. The large animal rotation segment dealt primarily with horses, pigs, cattle, sheep, and goats. One of my most memorable large animal rotation cases was "Mike", a four year old, big and powerful Clydesdale stallion. He was truly a gentle giant, if ever there was one. Mike was pitch black in color, with a white stripe down his forehead, and he had those long tufts of white hair, called feathers, above each hoof. He was a very handsome guy, and he knew it too. Mike was at the veterinary school hospital because of a medical problem that involved his left front hoof, and the treatment consisted of cleaning, medicating, and bandaging that enormous hoof twice daily. I was assigned to Mike's care during my two week rotation stint, and we became pretty good buddies over that extended period of time. Mike was a smart ombre, and had more than his share of that proverbial horse sense. He seemed to instinctively know when it was treatment time. He'd stand there with his big head draped over the paddock wall, eagerly eye-balling me as I approached. Mike was a good patient, —surprisingly easy to handle and lead, very cooperative, and he liked all the attention. I was extremely thankful too, because Mike stood over eighteen hands (about 6 feet) tall at the withers, weighed over 2,000 pounds, and had hooves the size of dinner plates. I'd get him cross-tied in the treatment stanchion, and attempt to get that huge, heavy hoof situated between my knees so it could be cleaned and treated. Believe me, I was in a vulnerable position, — and Mike knew it. He didn't struggle or object, —thank goodness, — but he was a trickster, and he couldn't resist nibbling on my ear, —sensing that I was in a compromised stance where I couldn't defend myself. As I was intently working on his hoof, I'd occasionally feel this delicate tickling sensation on my ear. It was from the small hairs on his muzzle. It's hard to believe that this huge, powerful horse, with a muzzle the size of an over inflated football, could be so gentle. I'd reach up with one hand and tap him on the muzzle while saying, "KNOCK IT OFF, MIKE". That only slowed him down for a minute or two, and then he was back at it again. He had that look in his eyes not unlike that of some mischievous little kid, —just annoying someone for the fun of it. I swear, there were times that it sounded like he was actually snickering. The treatment sessions took quite a while to complete, because it went something like this: — clean — swat — clean — tap — "knock it off, Mike", — clean — swat — etc. His hoof eventually healed, and when he went back home I honestly missed that big dude. One thing for sure, I thoroughly enjoyed working with Mike,— he was my Clydesdale buddy.

The Simplot Rotation

A nother of the clinical rotations, especially for those individuals who would be treating large animals in the future, was the two week block at the Simplot cattle ranch located in southern Idaho. The Simplot Company was involved in various business ventures, including potato production, feedlots, and cow-calf operations, just to name a few. We were to go to the cow-calf center, where about one thousand young cows and first calf heifers would be calving. Most of the cows were brought in directly from the range lands to the holding pens without having much prior exposure to humans. That made for a very interesting situation. The Simplot managers gave full permission to the third year veterinary students to perform any medical procedure necessary, including cesarians. It was a win-win deal, — Simplot got extra veterinary help, and we as eager students had an opportunity to gain invaluable hands-on experience.

Some of Simplot's hired hands included hardcore cowboys who looked and acted as if they'd just stepped out of the 1800's, and some Basques who provided care for the sheep primarily, but they also pitched in with the cattle. The chow hall was extremely clean, but spartan, — no frills! The menu was carefully planned to meet the high caloric requirements of a hard working crew, and the food was very tasty and plentiful. There were strict time schedules for meals, — you better not be late, — and there wasn't much time to sit and shoot the bull. It was strictly regimented, — eat quickly, —refuel, — and get back to work. We were essentially on call 24/7, and slept only when time permitted, — but it was a great experience, one which I'm grateful to have had.

Our duties were to assist with the calving. Some calves were coming backwards, i.e. posterior presentation, there were hip lock cases, breaches, uterine inertias wherein the muscles of the uterus fatigued and there were hardly any contractions, and we also did some caesarian section surgeries. The hours were long, but the experience was priceless! Many of the cowboys called us, "Doc", and that sounded good for a change. Even better, was earning the trust and confidence of the regular crew. On one particular occasion, there was a very wild Charlois cross cow standing out in the center of the large corral, with a calf dangling out of her with its hips locked tight in her pelvis. From a distance, the calf appeared alive, but we couldn't tell for sure because the cow wouldn't let anyone get close. Whenever someone attempted to direct her into one of the calving stalls, she'd snort, paw at the ground, bellow, and swing her head wildly in the air, — getting ready to charge. All the while the calf was swinging back and forth under her tail. The calf's position hadn't changed, and something needed to be done for that calf, and done quickly or else it would surely die. The smaller calving stalls were located on both sides of a long alley runway that was connected to the large open corral. Getting that wild cow down the runway and into one of those stalls would be pretty tricky. None of the guys had any solutions, — and then I chimed out, "I've got an idea!" You see, I'd grown up around cattle. I'd learned, by experience, how to read their body language, and how to react and respond to their moves. I'd been to the "school of hard knocks" — literally. Over the years I'd been charged, butted, kicked, run over, and horn whipped. I'd learned how to watch their eyes, how to time their charges, and I felt confident that I could get this wild cow into one of those holding stalls, — and come away clean! I wasn't intimidated or afraid of that cow, but I had a healthy respect for her and the damage she could potentially inflict. It was always an adrenaline rush to go one-on-one against a big charging animal, — really exhilarating! Believe me, my heart would really get a-pounding! It was exciting! I loved it!

I told the guys, "I'll go out there and approach her — she'll charge me, — and when she does, I'll run down the alley way, with her right on my tail, — I'll swing into one of the calving stalls, and get out by climbing over the rear wall (about 6 foot)." Everybody thought I was nuts, — but it seemed like a good plan to me. "Everybody ready?" I shouted. Then into the large holding corral I went. When the cow spotted me, she immediately swung her head high in the air, — blew snot, pawed the ground with her hooves, bellowed, — then lowered her head, and, — here she comes! —— RUN!!! I thought that I was doing pretty good until some of the guys yelled, "FASTER! – SHE'S GAINING ON YA!" I ran down the alley, made a quick turn into a stall, got my hands on the top board of the stall, and at that precise moment, the cow whipped her head and caught me square in the seat of my pants!. She launched me into the air, — up, out, and over the wall. It all happened in the blink of an eye. Then that deranged cow attempted to jump over the almost six foot tall enclosure, and in so doing, got temporarily hung up on the top board. The pressure on her abdomen and her frantic struggling caused the LIVE calf's hips to free up, and the calf fell to the ground. That maniacal cow eventually maneuvered herself over the wall, — high tailed it outa there, — and never looked back. — GONE!

Hey, — that was a wild experience, and a lot of fun too! I'd managed to escape with only a few bruises, and on the positive side, we'd found a new and novel method to free up a hip locked calf!

13

The Next Step

Those first three years of vet school had gone by in a flash. Here I was, in my final year, and almost ready to go out into the real world as a full-fledged veterinarian. It was almost unbelievable. The past three years had been intense, stressful, and also humbling. Many sacrifices had been made to get to this point in our lives, yet we would have gladly done it all over again. We didn't have much money during those college years, so we were forced to live very frugally. Our dining out consisted of going to the local drive-in once a month for the five burgers for $1.00 special. We also splurged on a small side of fries and one milkshake. I had two of the cardboard burgers, while Sandy and our four-year-old son, Eric, shared the remaining three. The greasy fries were a real treat, and Eric thoroughly enjoyed the runny shake. Hey, we were happy and didn't realize how poor we really were. Our entertainment was simple and, most importantly, affordable. We didn't have a TV, so we listened to the radio, went for walks, sang songs, took short trips to nearby Kamiak Butte for day hikes, and went to the pig barns to watch the little piglets scurry all over the place. They were really funny! Believe me, those times of simple pleasures and cheap entertainment provided us with many fond memories.

Then the time came to carefully think about finding employment after graduation. That was a new and exciting thought, considering the fact that I'd been a student for the last eight years. All the senior vet students would make their daily pilgrimage to the jobs board to peruse the latest posting of employment opportunities. There were positions available in all kinds of practices from all over the country. You could actually choose where you wanted to live and work. It was such a different concept to realize that you were about to enter a medical profession that was in demand and that the days of looking for part-time summer work was over.

There was one particular posting that seemed to appeal to me more than the others. It was a veterinary practice located in a smaller town near Mount Rainier. It was a mixed practice, meaning, veterinary services were provided for both large and small animal, and there were many dairy operations in the area as well. I wrote down the telephone number of the veterinary clinic from the posting and was anxious to contact the practice and find out if the position was still available. When I got home from school that day, I said to Sandy, "How would you like to live near Mount Rainier?" She quickly replied, "How close?" I told her that I didn't know, but I'd find out.

This was starting to get exciting! I proceeded to make the call, talked to the veterinarian, and we set up a time for an interview. The name of the town was Enumclaw, population about five thousand, located near Crystal Mountain Ski Resort, and surrounded by several smaller communities. It sounded like a great place to live and work. Looking at the map, we saw that Enumclaw was located at the base of Chinook Pass, not far from the larger neighboring city of Auburn. So far, so good.

The interview, with Dr. Wagner went very well. He was enthusiastic, congenial, easy to talk to, and I felt comfortable with the relationship. Dr. Wagner must have had the same impression because he offered me the position of associate veterinarian at the Enumclaw Veterinary Clinic. I accepted, sight unseen. Sandy was extremely excited too and we decided to make a weekend trip over the mountains to actually see this community that would become our future home. The weather was absolutely stunning the day of our trip. The clear blue sky and gentle warm breezes made the drive over to Western Washington very enjoyable. We took an exit from I-90, headed south on Highway 18, turned left on Highway 169. The forest of tall dark-green cedar trees stood as silent sentinels, hugging and dwarfing the road leading to Enumclaw. Suddenly, as we rounded a bend in the road, there it stood in all its glory, *the* mountain, Mount Rainier. There wasn't a cloud in the sky, and that majestic snow-capped mountain stood directly in the center of the road, framed by the towering cedars. That sight was absolutely breathtaking. It made a person so very thankful just to be alive and to be able to experience such beauty.

As we drove by the numerous dairy farms and smaller ranches with horses and dogs running about, it became quite evident that veterinary services were really needed here. When finally arriving in Enumclaw, I told Sandy, "I think we made the right decision. I *know* we made the right decision."

INTO THE FRAY

Hey, Doc

Rumbling down the road with all of our belongings packed into the back of the cattle truck made us strangely resemble the "Beverly Hillbillies". What can I say, it worked, and the price was right. We lucked out that day, because the weather was good, —no rain. There we were, on our way to a new town, and me starting my career as a veterinarian. The whole experience seemed almost unreal. A dream, along with a lot of effort and willing sacrifice, had finally come true. We were filled with excitement and anticipation of what the future had in store for us, and there were plenty of butterflies in our stomachs as well, especially mine, trying to grasp all the major changes that were rapidly impacting our lives.

My first day as a practicing veterinarian was unlike anything that I'd expected. Instead of jumping directly into the fray, I was given a short introduction to the countryside, and the overall thrust of the practice. I was to observe the way things were done. The practice was extremely busy, phones ringing incessantly and staff scurrying about frantically in preparation for the day's schedule of activity. I quickly learned that they were shorthanded. The previous associate veterinarian had moved on, and Dr. Wagner, the owner, had been the sole veterinarian for quite some time now, and was in dire need of some relief. It appeared to me that the workload of the practice could easily keep three veterinarians busy, — so, — nothing like jumping right into the fire. I accompanied Dr. Wagner on his rounds that first day, taking notes on all the different roads, medications and treatments used, and how to charge for services rendered. Believe me, it was like mental overload, big time! Dr. Wagner told me, "Don't worry. You'll get the hang of it in no time." Over the next couple weeks I became familiar with the area, the people, and the practice. One day, I noticed an old beat-up portable medical case called a "Pandora Box" setting next to the garbage can at the rear of the clinic. It was all scuffed up, had hinges missing, and some of the compartments were damaged and displaced. It looked pretty sad. I knew that those boxes were quite expensive, and I'd always wanted to purchase one, but couldn't afford paying the price. I asked Dr. Wagner why the Pandora Box was sitting by the garbage can. Dr. Wagner answered, "It's junk! It's seen its better days. It's been dropped, stepped on, — and into, crapped on, and the goats have even tried to eat it. It's going into file 13." I asked him, "Can I have it?" "Sure, if you want it, it's yours." Came the reply. It has been said that beauty is in the eye of the beholder, and my previous eight years of poverty had taught me how to make a silk purse out of a sow's ear. As I feasted my eyes on that old dilapidated box, — I could see that it had definite possibilities. So, down to the hardware store I went, bought hinges, tape, and black shoe polish, — hoping to resurrect my newly acquired prized possession. It's truly amazing what a little sweat equity and some ingenuity can accomplish. Dr. Wagner just laughed and shook his head when he saw how good that ole beat-up box looked after I'd performed my magic on it. That restored Pandora Box served me well for over ten years.

I arrived at the clinic at little early the next morning, partly because of excitement, but I also needed to prepare myself for the coming events of the day. Roberta, the receptionist/assistant was already there, but Dr. Wagner hadn't yet arrived, — so I thought. "What time does Dr. Wagner get in?" I inquired. "Oh, he's not coming in today, because he really needs some time off. He's been going at it pretty hard since the other vet left, and now he really needs a break. He deserves it." Roberta retorted. Then she said, "You're it!". Momentary panic and an overwhelming sense of responsibility hit me all at the same time. "You need to be here, then there, by 10 AM, so get the surgeries done quickly, and be ready for emergencies." She added. I told myself, "Focus, — just stay focused! Don't make any mistakes. Eat on the run. Don't get lost on the farm calls. Get through the cases, even if it takes all day and most of the night." So, — this is what it was REALLY like being a veterinarian in a busy practice. It was fun, challenging, and at times, physically and mentally exhausting. But, through it all, being addressed with, "Hey, Doc", made it all worthwhile.

A Valuable Lesson

Walking into the clinic each morning was not unlike being announced as the "Blue Light" special. I was greeted with, "Get ready Doc, its going to be a wild and bumpy one today." One quick glance at the handwritten schedule of booked and double booked appointments verified Roberta's prophetic statement. Strangely missing was "lunch". Was that just an accidental omission, — or was she really serious? The way things were to turn out that day, — she was serious.

The first surgical case of the day was an ovariohysterectomy (spay) on an eight month old white cat named "Pinkie". She was a good little girl, purred constantly, and seemed overly affectionate, — rubbing her head against everything and everybody. These not-so-subtle amorous marking cues suggested that Pinkie was very possibly in heat. If she were, then the uterine tissues would be much more delicate and fragile, —requiring extra care and caution during surgery. Pinkie was anesthetized, prepped, and readied for surgery. The initial abdominal incision was made, and the uterus along with the ovaries were quickly isolated. The uterus was slightly enlarged, there were follicles plainly visible on the ovaries, and the adjacent blood vessels also appeared larger. The verdict, — this little lady was in roaring heat, — and I'd need some additional assistance to retract the delicate uterus while placing the ligatures. So, I called out to Roberta for some help, "Roberta, could you please come and retract for me?" — No response. I called out again, only this time with more volume and urgency.

25

Finally, — a disgruntled Roberta appeared. "Why can't you do this yourself? Dr. Wagner doesn't ever need help." "Roberta," I said. "Dr. Wagner has about fifteen more years of experience than me, — and after a few more of these, I won't need any help either, — but for now, I need an extra hand, — OK!" I explained the delicate tissue concern and the extra care needed, but it obviously went in one ear and out the other, because when I gently handed the forceps, which were attached to the uterus, to Roberta, she jerked up on them abruptly in disgust. The fragile tissue instantly snapped, causing the body of the uterus and the adjacent vessels to plunge back down into the recesses of the abdominal cavity. There was immediate panic! Roberta's face turned pale, and she was speechless, — for a change. I could feel my chest tighten and my heart rate increase, — sensing the gravity of what had just happened. Pinkie could possibly bleed internally if I couldn't quickly find the uterine stump and vessels and tie them off. I enlarged the incision for better exposure, and to my amazement, there was no bleeding. The quick jerk on the fragile tissue had caused the vessels to constrict, and stopped any potential hemorrhaging. I did find the vessels and tied them off, just to avoid any further complications. Pinkie recovered very nicely, and went home the next day, — happy and none the worse for wear.

The whole incident was an extremely valuable lesson for both Roberta and myself. She never again questioned my request for assistance. She also became a more gentle, proficient, and compassionate assistant, and I'd learned how to effectively respond in high stress, life threatening situations. That experience was a real adrenaline rush, but more importantly, — the patient survived and was doing well.

New Medicine

A s I walked into the clinic that morning, our receptionist, Roberta, greeted me with, "Hey, Doc, you've got to go out to Van Leeuwen's place today. He's got a cow that he thinks has mastitis, and he says her bag is hot and pretty big and hard too. Don't try to get him to use penicillin on any of his cows because he doesn't believe in the stuff. Oh yeah, and don't even try to get him to come into the clinic, for anything, because Dr. Wagner has tried that for years, and Sam has never come in, ever."

The ole Dutch dairyman, Sam Van Leeuwen, sounded like a real character and a challenge. I was actually looking forward to going on this farm call and meeting Sam. You see, I grew up in an ethnically German community, heard farmers and ranchers converse a lot in German, and I'd experienced the stubbornness of some of those people and how they could be firmly set in their ways. Believe me, I'd seen firsthand how change was hard for many of them to accept. Heck, dealing with ole Sam would be like "old home week." It sounded like fun!

Driving through the countryside on the way to Sam's place was great. The scenery was a real feast for the eyes, especially on that nice day with the sun shining down on all the cattle and horses grazing contentedly on the pastures. Once in a while, I'd get a perfect view of snow-capped Mount Rainier towering majestically in the distance. It was a sight to behold. I definitely understood why people had chosen to live and work in this part of the country.

My sightseeing ventured ended as I pulled up to the Van Leeuwen dairy farm. It wasn't a large operation, but dairies didn't have to be big to be good. Suddenly a skinny little man dressed in overalls, wearing black barn boots, and sporting an old misshapen baseball cap came marching out from one of the white barns. He waved an arm in the air with a welcoming gesture and approached my vehicle. "*Wie gehts*, Sam," I said, hoping he could understand my German greeting. Sam replied with a wry smile, "*Gute*." Well, that was a good ice breaker. So far, so good. "*You da nu Dokk?*" he asked. "*Ja, Ich bin der tierarzt.*" (Yes, I am the animal doctor, veterinarian.) "I understand that you've got a cow with udder problems. Is that right? "*Ja*, her bag is hot, and dere's some blud in da mielk too."

Sam led the way to the barn, and I followed close behind with my stainless-steel bucket in one hand and the medical bag in the other. I examined the cow, and Sam was right on the money with his diagnosis. The cow's rectal temperature was elevated, her udder was swollen, discolored, very warm to the touch, and when I stripped milk from one of the teats, it was bloody, thick, and stringy. I told Sam that his cow did indeed have a bad case of mastitis, and I had a "new," very special mastitis medicine with me that I wanted to use on his cow. I had taken a brand-new bottle of penicillin, added 2 cc of azosulfamide solution, which was deep red in color, mixed the contents, and – voila! – the "new Medicine." I reached into my medicine bag, grabbed the unlabeled pink concoction, showed it to Sam, and told him, "I'll give the cow an injection of this new medicine now, and if it appears to work, then you'll have to come to the clinic and pick up another syringe of the stuff, okay?"

Sam nodded his head in agreement. As I was about to leave, I told him that I was pretty confident that this new mastitis treatment would help. Deep down inside, I knew it would. Now the big question, could I get Same to show up at the clinic – something he'd never done before? Time would tell.

Three days later, Roberta came rushing back into the clinic treatment area, and with a shocked expression on her face, she said, "You'll never believe who just walked into the clinic. Sam Van Leeuwen, and he wants to see... YOU! How'd you do that?" Looking nonchalantly at Roberta, I said, "A trade secret." Oh yeah, the treatment on Sam's cow was a success, and in time, his confidence in the healing power of penicillin was restored.

A pastoral view of Mt. Rainier

That Was Fast!

Holstein cows tend to be very large animals, and when they have problems, those problems can be rather big too. Such was the case with Lawrence Purdy's cow. There were numerous dairy farms in the Enumclaw area. Various breeds of cattle were used for milk production, including the Jerseys, Guernseys, and Holsteins. The Jersey cows were smaller in stature, but they had those big beautiful dark eyes and the extra long black eyelashes. As far as cows go, — they were, in my humble opinion, the prettiest. Holstein cows, on the other hand, were something quite the opposite. It's not unusual to find a mature Holstein cow that tips the scales at between 1,500 and 2,000 pounds, stands over 5 feet tall at the shoulders, and is close to 3 feet across the hips. These gals are big, and so are their parts, — both inside and out.

The drive to Mr. Purdy's dairy that morning was enjoyable. As I passed by the numerous wild blackberry patches alongside the road, the sun began to peek out between the clouds that had brought rain earlier that morning. The sky was blue, the air was clean and clear, and the sun was shining, —— "This should be a wonderful day", I said to myself as I entered Mr. Purdy's driveway.

This dairy was one of the largest in the area. The out buildings and barns appeared well maintained, suggesting that the owner was very conscientious and took pride in his work. I pulled into the farmyard and stopped my truck at the exact moment that Mr. Purdy emerged from one of the barns. He walked up to the truck, saw me, and said, "He didn't send me another "newbie" again, did he?" Mr. Purdy appeared and sounded disgusted. I stretched forth my hand and introduced myself, "I'm Dr. Roloff, — Dr. Wagner's new associate." Mr. Purdy ignored my handshake, looked to the side and said, "Yeah,— that's what I thought. He always sends me somebody who's green. Well, you're all I got, — so, — it's this way to the cow, — she prolapsed her uterus. I knew, right then and there, that this was going to be a tough case, and there'd be a lot of equipment and medications to carry to the barn. I asked, "Mr. Purdy, — could you help me carry some of this stuff?" He opened the gate, and just kept walking, not looking back. I wasn't sure if he heard me, or if he was just being rude, disgusted, and ignored my request. Anyway, there I was, buckets and ropes in one hand, and portable medical case in the other, — shutting the gates with my shoulders and feet. I sure could have used some help, — but didn't get any. As I entered the barn, — there she stood! This huge, behemoth of a cow with her uterus totally prolapsed. Gads! Reducing (replacing) this uterus would be a long and difficult task, — that was for sure. As I proceeded to clean the bloody, swollen, edematous, straw-covered mass of tissue, I heard Mr. Purdy comment, "I suppose we'll be here almost all day, because it takes Doc Wagner a couple hours to do these, — and he's good." Boy, that was sure a confidence builder! I didn't respond to his put down, instead, I just kept on doing my job. I then gave the cow an epidural anesthetic to decrease the cow's straining, and to make the whole replacement procedure easier on both of us. That pendulous uterus weighed almost 70 pounds, was about two feet wide, and hung down over half way to her hocks. Attempting to push something that big back into a 1,500 pound cow, through a small opening, while she was still straining in resistance, was definitely not going to be a walk in the park. All the while, Mr. Purdy was standing silently to the side with an "I knew it" smirk on his face. As I grunted to get the weighty uterus into position, suddenly

I felt the tissue beginning to involute (turn in on itself), — and that was the key. The use of steady even force allowed the the uterus to magically fold in on itself, and in the blink of an eye, the mass tumbled completely back into its normal position. Quite honestly, — I was shocked. — It was a minor miracle! I wanted that thing to stay put, so I placed a few temporary restraining sutures (stitches), gave her several antibiotic injections, and I was done! — It took less than 10 minutes! I nonchalantly looked over at Mr. Purdy with a cheshire cat smile on my face. His mouth was hanging wide open, and he looked as if he'd just seen a ghost. "How'd you do that so fast?" He asked. Very calmly and without smiling, I said. "If you know what you're doing, it should always work like that." Mr. Purdy was speechless! I grabbed my buckets and equipment, handed them to Mr. Purdy, and told him, "Now, — here,— carry my stuff to the truck." Without a moments hesitation, the stunned Mr. Purdy grabbed the buckets, and even managed to open the gates for me as we returned to the truck. His demeanor had suddenly become much more civil. He actually seemed appreciative and somewhat humbled, but more likely, he was in a state of shock and disbelief at what he'd just witnessed.

I couldn't stop smiling on the drive back to the vet clinic, because replacing a prolapsed uterus on a cow that big,— that fast, was almost unbelievable. I'd definitely been graced out. — Thank you, Lord. Hey, — the day really did turn out to be beautiful, — in more ways than one.

The Gray Stallion

Being a veterinarian in a mixed practice was never boring or mundane. It was exciting going to work each day, anticipating what interesting cases lay ahead. Most days were, as Forrest Gump put it, "like a box of chocolates. You don't know what you are going to get." Truer words were never spoken.

"Doc, you got to get out to Milton Stables. They've got a horse that hurt his mouth."

"Is that it? They didn't tell you anymore?" I asked. Roberta curtly replied, "Nope."

I grabbed what I thought I'd need to handle just about anything. Heck, the horse could have an abscessed tooth, or maybe he had bitten himself, or his teeth might need to be floated – all kinds of things could be going on here. I'd just have to wait and see. Milton Stables was a top-class equine breeding operation. White wooden fences flanked the long entry lane that led up to the headquarters atop a grassy knoll.

There were numerous white and green barns surrounded by various-sized separation pens. White fences were everywhere, and it all appeared perfectly manicured. Well-groomed horses were all about, whinnying in delight as they ran and jumped around in their corrals. It looked like something you'd expect to see in an oil painting. The foreman approached. I introduced myself and asked to see the horse with a mouth problem. He led me over to a small corral where the big, muscular, gray quarter horse stallion was busily eating grass hay. I thought to myself, *He's eating, so this shouldn't be too bad.* That's what I thought until the foreman turned the horse's head toward me.

"Holy cow." I said. "His jaw is broken."

"Yup," the foreman responded. "I shouldn't have put those two stallions so close together. They're always fighting over the mares and trying to bite each other through the fence. Something must've happened.

No kidding, I thought to myself. The horse didn't seem to be in much pain or discomfort, and that in itself was amazing. His lower jaw was totally split in half, and the now separated jaw bones moved freely and independently. "This horse needs surgery, and pronto!" I told the foreman.

Thank goodness the weather was cooperating. The day was warm, sunny, and best of all, no rain. I placed the horse under general anesthetic on the lawn atop the grassy knoll. As I opened the horse's mouth, the lower jaw separated approximately four inches. What a mess! The symphysis, the union point of the right and left sides of the lower jaw, was completely split. Pieces of grass and plant seed were stuck into the exposed porous openings of the bone marrow. All the debris had to be painstakingly removed to prevent a severe bone infection from occurring. Once the cleaning of the tissues had been completed, I wired the horse's jaw back into place with some very stout stainless steel surgical wire and reconstructed the soft tissue. Upon completion, it looked really good, almost as if nothing had happened.

The stainless steel wires would stay for eight to ten weeks. Antibiotics were to be given, and my final instructions: *keep those stallions apart!* He did, and the big, gray stallion did just fine.

She's So Small

Why do emergencies always seem to happen at the most inopportune times? The unspoken code in the medical profession is, "You Must Attend", — but what does that really mean? It essentially means that you drop whatever you're presently doing, and immediately address the problem at hand. Such was the case on one particular Saturday evening.

The caseload had been pretty hectic the last few weeks, and I was seriously in need of a break. That Saturday morning's appointments were basically routine cases, fairly easy stuff, — no major problems to deal with. I was looking forward to getting off at noon, but was scheduled to be on call that evening. Saturday evenings were usually rather quiet, so Sandy and I thought we'd treat ourselves by going out to dinner at one of the local restaurants. We definitely needed and deserved some quiet, relaxed time together.

It was 7:30 P.M., — and just as we were about to leave on our dinner date, — the phone rang. "I hope it isn't what I think it is." Sandy said as she picked up the receiver. She stood there, listening for a minute or so, then said, "Here's Doc.", and handed me the phone. I listen to the concerned owner, — told him that I'd be right out, and hung up the phone. I turned to Sandy and dejectedly said, "The guy on the phone has a first calf heifer that's been straining hard for several hours, trying to deliver a calf, but nothing's happened. — I'm so sorry Dear, but I've gotta go. I'm on call, and small, first calf heifers usually have more trouble calving, and those difficult births can be life threatening to the cow, the calf, or both of them. It sounds like a bona fide emergency, — and I might end up doing a c-section tonight.— I guess we'll have to take a rain-check on that dinner date." Sandy, bless her heart, said, "That's alright. Would you mind if I came along?" I told her, "That would be great". Sandy had never seen a caesarian section performed on a cow, so this would be a first. She was a nurse by profession, and she was willing to pitch in and help if I needed assistance. We quickly changed clothes,— because now we were headed out on a "dystocia" (difficult birthing) date — instead of a dinner date.

The small farm was located on the edge of town, so it didn't take long to get there. The hobby farmer and his wife were standing by their driveway, awaiting our arrival, and were extremely grateful that we'd come to their aid, especially on a Saturday evening. As we entered the barn, — there she stood. —— Undeniably the smallest Hereford first calf heifer that I'd ever seen! That diminutive little girl had c-section written all over her, — no doubt about it. "What was she bred to?" I asked. "A Hereford bull." The man responded. Oh joy! — Hereford bulls usually produce big calves, — and that could create some problems. I got all my buckets, disinfectants, medications, and surgical instruments prepared and organized together, — anticipating a c-section, but first I needed to examine the heifer and check the position of the calf, and also see if the calf was still alive. As I inserted my arm into the birth canal, I palpated (felt) a very small hoof, — it was tiny, — like that of a fawn. "That's strange", I thought. Then the little hoof pulled back. "It's ALIVE and SMALL!" I announced. "I might be able to deliver this little guy". I aligned the little calf's legs, and as I applied steady, even traction, the heifer strained and forcefully contracted her abdominal muscles, — groaning with each heavy contraction. I grabbed ahold of the hooves, and synchronized my pulling with her contractions. First came the tiny hooves, — then the nose appeared, — next, the head popped out of the birth canal, — and finally the body was exposed. It took only a bit more traction and the little fella was delivered. At first the calf laid motionless, but after some vigorous rubbing and tickling its nose, — the little guy blinked his dark brown eyes, coughed, took a deep breath, and then forcefully blew fluid out of his little pink nose. When the calf belted out its first bleat, — the little cow turned and immediately started vigorously licking her baby calf all over its head and body with her raspy tongue. She was a good "Mom", and she was sure proud and protective of that calf too.

As they say, "All's well that ends well". What could have been a disaster, turned out to be something extra special and meaningful. We'd witnessed the miracle of birth, and it's a wonderful experience, — each and every time. "Hey Sandy, — we've still got some time tonight. Let's go home, get cleaned up, go out to dinner —— and CELEBRATE!

Pasture Cowboy

S ecretly, I'd always wanted to be a rodeo clown. Having a 2000 pound animal charging you, intending to put your lights out, is an adrenalin rush like no other. Escaping unharmed and in one piece was definitely a thrill.

I had what might be called an easy farm call to go on that morning. — Just one bull calf to castrate at Mr. Corless's place. Heck, that shouldn't take any time at all, so I thought. The directions were good, so it didn't take much time to get there. Instead of a farm, it turned out to be a 30 acre pasture with a small herd of cattle grazing in the far corner, and a little red barn sitting next to the road. I got out of my vet rig, looked around, — no vehicles, — nothin. It was as quiet as a tomb. I called out, "Hello, anybody here? Mr. Corless, – are you here?" – No answer. — Where was everybody? Where was Mr. Corless? Did I screw up on the directions? I waited for a few more minutes, and then decided to take off. Suddenly, just as I was about to leave, a short, pudgy, elderly gent dressed in bib overalls and wearing a long sleeved red and black colored plaid shirt, materialized out from behind the barn. It was Mr. Corless. He approached with a waddling shuffle, waving his arm in the air, — letting me know that he was on his way. When he got within earshot, I introduced myself and asked, "Where's the calf that needs to be castrated?" I'd surmised that the calf was pinned up and waiting for me in the barn, but Mr. Corless motioned his arm in the direction of the pasture. "Out there?" I asked. He nodded yes, not speaking, and seemingly out of breath. Mr. Corless looked to be in his eighty's, and by the way he was breathing, not in the best of health either. Looking around, there didn't appear to be anything that resembled a corral or catch area for confining the calf. Nothing, – nada, – zippo! Mr. Corless then told me, "He's out there with the cows." "What kind of cows do you have, and how many?" I asked. "Simmentals, — twelve cows and just one bull calf, – about 200 pounds." He replied. Now, Simmentals are an old breed of cattle that originated from Switzerland. They are big, heavily muscled, and were used primarily for milk production and drafting (pulling wagons and plows). Simmentals usually stand about 5 feet tall at the withers, and can weigh nearly 1500 pounds when mature. They also have huge muzzles, about the width of a good sized cantaloupe. Simmentals are a gentle breed of cattle, but can be very protective of their young, which is normal.

Mr. Corless then popped the big question that I really didn't want to hear, "You gotta rope?" I had a lariat in the vet rig, and unfortunately it looked like I'd be using my roping skills, which in all honesty, weren't very good. The challenge now was, how can I get to the calf that's way out there in the pasture surrounded by twelve protective cows? There I was, a stranger with a lariat draped over my shoulder, carrying a clanging bucket of surgical instruments, invading their territory. The cows immediately sensed danger, and with their heads raised in alarm position, they started stampeding from one end of the pasture to the other. The calf, all the while, was being surrounded by the protective cows, and my approaching moves caused the small herd to run off in panic mode. I noticed that the herd seemed to run in a circular pattern, so I strategically positioned myself, hoping for a closer run-by. Suddenly and unexpectedly, the thundering herd came my way, and I got a glimpse of the calf. — Here was my big chance. I swung the rope over my head, took a sizable lead, and blindly tossed the lariat in the general direction of the calf. Amazingly, as the lariat reached it's full extention, the calf's head miraculously passed perfectly through the loop. I leaned back on the rope as the loop tightened around the calf's neck, — ya know, the way real cowboys do it. GOT HIM! The calf lost his balance, fell to the ground and let out a loud bellow alarm for help. The cows immediately answered the call and came rushing to his rescue, — and at that very moment, I knew it was, — now or never! I had to get to the calf quickly, hold on for dear life, and hopefully not get trampled by those 1500 pound cows trying to save one of their own. As long as I held onto the calf, I was semi-safe, because the cows didn't want to hurt their calf, — just me! I tied up three of the calf's legs in a flash, grabbed the bucket containing the surgical instruments, and performed the fastest castration ever, —— probably record setting time! All the while, the frantic, protective cows were literally on top of me, — bellowing directly into my ears, and flinging slobber from their huge muzzles all over my head and shoulders. As I untied the rope, the calf made his great escape and the cows reassuringly followed. My ears were still ringing as I stumbled to my feet. Out of the corner of my eye, I noticed Mr. Corless shuffling along through the pasture in my direction. Although visibly tired and out of breath, he still managed to ask, "Doc, ya need any help?" I replied, "Nah, my cowboy'n is done. I only wish somebody could have timed that castration, and given me a score on my calf roping time."

He or She?

The phrase, "one in a million", usually congers up thoughts of winning the lottery or having someone ring your doorbell announcing that you'd just won the big sweepstakes. Well, this one particular day would be a "one in a million" day, but not the kind where money was involved.

"Doc, a lady just called and she wants you to check out something that's growing by her dog's private parts." Roberta, the receptionist, loudly announced from the front desk. "She said it looks weird, and just noticed it yesterday. Whatcha think it is?" "I don't know. It could be a lot of things. We'll just have to wait and see. "I said. We didn't have to wait long, because the owner considered the growth to be an emergency, and was rushing right in.

The fifteen pound, brown and white Terrier cross, intact female named "Lilly" arrived and was quickly placed on the exam table. She was visibly nervous, very wary of the surroundings, and was repeatedly licking at her, "parts". "Let's take a look." I said while lifting her tail. There it was for all the world to see. The owner was right. A cylindrical shaped growth, the size of a person's little finger, was protruding from Lilly's vulva. The tissue appeared to be pink and healthy, but definitely in the wrong place. Upon closer examination, the unusual growth appeared to be a vestigial (rudimentary, undeveloped, nonfunctional) penis. "We could have a little hermaphrodite or pseudo-hermaphrodite here." I told the owner. "I'll need to surgically remove that growth and also perform a spay at the same time, because there could be some associated ovary problems as well." I then asked the owner if she had ever noticed Lilly acting more like a male than a female. Does Lilly squat or hike her leg when she urinates? The owner replied, "She always hikes her leg, and humps the pillows too. — Isn't that bizarre for a female? "Yup, and it could indicate that there might be some additional problems inside of her too. You see, the sex of an individual, whether they're male or female, is determined by the gonad (ovary or testicle) that is present, — not the external plumbing. Lilly could have one or the other, or both, — as is the case with a true hermaphrodite. We'll see." I said.

The surgery was quickly scheduled. The vestigial penis was removed and an ovariohystectomy (spay) was performed. Lilly did have a normal uterus, but instead of ovaries, she had testicles in the place where the ovaries should have been. So, Lilly was technically a male! — a boy! —a guy! Following the surgery, I delicately dissected free, and surgically removed the vestigial penis. It contained a bony structure called the os penis,— which is a normal structure found in male dogs. I cleaned it real well and took it home, — hoping to someday make it into a tie tac. That would make a conversation piece like no other! When Sandy saw my souvenir, she couldn't believe that I'd actually brought that "thing" home, and she thought my tie tac idea was gross and weird.—— So, she threw it in the garbage without me knowing. When I found out that my little trophy was long gone, I was bummed out, because I'd most likely never see another case like that,— ever again in my lifetime. It was an extremely rare, — one in a million find, — now gone. Oh well, c'est la vie.

Lilly had to be renamed because she turned out to be more of a boy than a girl. So, instead of Lilly, — HE became "Lawrence", even though he still had female/girl external plumbing.

The Forbidden Fruit

Stan Winslow, a commercial airline pilot who flew out of Seattle's Seatac Airport, loved the Pacific Northwest, and had made Enumclaw his home base. His small ranch of 50 acres served as his retreat from the hectic demands he routinely faced, and he found solace working with his small herd of twenty purebred Angus cows. He was, what you might call, a weekend rancher. Mr. Winslow dearly loved his cows, providing them with the best feed available and plenty of other goodies, including whole apples.

The caseload was comfortably slow that morning at the veterinary clinic. It was, undeniably, a welcomed change of pace. Everything was going along well, fairly routine cases, until the phone rang and Roberta said, "DOC, WE'VE GOT AN EMERGENCY! Stan Winslow is on the line and one of his cows is choking. You've got to get out there RIGHT NOW!" I quickly grabbed my stuff, and as I was racing out of the building, I yelled back to Roberta, "Reschedule whatever you can. — I'm outa here."

On the way to an emergency, I usually put the pedal to the metal, hoping not to get stopped by the police and having to explain myself. As I turned onto the lane leading up to Mr. Winslow's place, I could see him standing there with the choking cow, in a small pasture next to the house. The cow had her head extended down and forward, thrusting her tongue out as far as it could possibly go. She was heaving her chest and abdomen in a frantic attempt to dislodge whatever was in her throat, and it appeared that she wasn't getting any air either. No time for trying to find the mouth speculum that would keep her from biting me. I jumped out of the truck, ran over to the cow, and thrust my hand and arm into her mouth and down her throat, hoping to grab or dislodge whatever was causing the obstruction problem. All the while, this big panicking animal was chewing on my arm. At first I couldn't feel anything in her throat, but then as I thrust my arm deeper, to the point where the cow's muzzle was almost up to my shoulder, the tips of my fingers contacted a hard round object. It was positioned at the junction between the trachea (windpipe) and the esophagus, — essentially shutting off the air flow. It was too far down and too tightly wedged for me to grasp with my fingers, so my only option was to attempt to push it forward, — hoping she would swallow it. I flicked my fingers at the object while trying to thrust my chewed arm even deeper. Suddenly, IT MOVED forward, the cow swallowed hard several times, and then she took in a huge deep breath of air. That had to be one of the most beautiful sounds I'd ever heard. I quickly jerked my slobbery, bruised, chewed up arm out of that chomping cavern, and was thankful to see that I still had an arm. No more straining or choking as the cow wandered off. The cow and Mr. Winslow were both relieved, — and believe me, so was I. Honestly, I couldn't have taken much more, and neither could the cow.

"We dodged a bullet, Stan." I said. He shook his head in agreement. "you know, those whole apples are forbidden fruit to those cows, but if you're going to give them apples, cut them up into smaller pieces. — OK!" Mr. Winslow nodded sheepishly, and promised to feed only CUT UP apples in the future. It took several days for my arm to stop aching and heal.

The Devil's Rope

The expression, "good fences make good neighbors", is basically true, but fences are often like a two-edged sword in that they can either be a blessing or a curse. I've seen both ends of the spectrum, — especially where barbed wire was involved.

Barbed wire came on the scene in the late 1800's, changed the wild west, and is widely used throughout the world today. Why? — Because it's cheap, and very effective at setting boundaries. The flipside, however, is much more sinister. Those thin, spiked, twisted strands of metal wire are nearly invisible, and can pose a serious physical threat to any unsuspecting animal or human who unfortunately runs into or through it.

I was scheduled to work that Saturday morning, and it was also my turn to be "on call" for any weekend emergencies. It'd been a wild week at the clinic, — I was a little on the tired side, and needed a lighter weekend so I could recoup. The cases at the clinic that morning had been pretty routine, and it looked like I'd actually get out of there on time for a change. Wow! Wonders never cease! When I got home, Sandy greeted me with a neatly written "honey-do" list. That wasn't what I'd envisioned for the weekend, but at least it was a change of pace from what I'd been through the previous week.

All was going well until that 3:00 P.M. phone call. "Hello! This is Bonnie Calvert out here on 416th. — My horse just ran through some barbed wire. — He's cut up really bad on his chest and legs.— He's bleeding all over the place. — Can you come out right now? — Please!" I got directions, — grabbed my stuff, and kissed the honey-do list goodbye. — then hit the road. The Calvert place was located just a few miles outside of town, so I didn't have much time to conjure up a game plan. Usually I'd try to visualize what might be waiting for me, and get mentally prepared for what I was in for. Most of the time, however, things turned out to be much worse and more complicated than imagined, — and as I'd soon find out, that would also be the case in this instance. As I pulled into the Calvert's lane, there he stood. — A big, red roan quarter horse, surrounded by four women. One on the lead rope, trying to control the fidgety, stressed out horse, and the other three holding blood soaked towels to the horse's chest and upper front legs. The first thing I heard when getting out of the truck was, "Boy,— are we glad to see YOU!" As the women repositioned the towels, I got a quick glimpse at the barbed wire injuries, and instantly understood their reason for concern. — The horse was ripped to shreds! — Literally! This horse hadn't just been cut, — he'd been dissected!

The horse, named "Sid", was in obvious pain and discomfort, so I immediately gave him an injection containing a strong sedative and pain killer before proceeding any further. Once he was in La-La land and feeling no pain, I gently lifted the towels, quickly clamped the active bleeders, and surveyed the extent of tissue damage. There were multiple, traumatic lacerations to Sid's chest and upper front legs. The skin was savagely torn, and several lacerations had penetrated deeply into his chest muscles, completely severing some of the muscles, causing them to hang limply, almost half way down to his knees. As the saying goes, "First things first". I began by strategically injecting local anesthetic throughout the mangled mess, and then started the arduous task of cleaning, scrubbing, and disinfecting the surgical field prior to reconstruction. It was a challenge to identify what was what, and what went where. I mentally visualized the normal anatomical configuration of the muscles, and then began the painstakingly slow process of identifying and reuniting the muscles and reconstructing the severely damaged tissue. It took about two hours of intense surgery to put Sid back together, but when finished, I was confident that all the skin and muscles were successfully reunited, and I truly believed that he had a good chance of someday running again. Granted, Sid may have looked like an equine version of Frankenstein after the surgery, but it was now just a matter of time for complete healing to take place. — Time would tell.

When all the sutures were removed two weeks later, Sid looked and acted as good as new. He did run again, but had some permanent trophy scars as evidence of his untimely encounter with, "The Devil's Rope".

Moonshine

Black Diamond is a small town near Enumclaw, and an old mining cart is proudly displayed at one end of town. The town obviously derived its name from the mining of coal which was once a thriving industry in the area. At one time, coal miners from the Southeastern states ventured to the Pacific Northwest in search of work. Their immigration into the region gave rise to some neighboring villages and hamlets with names like Ravensdale, Carbonado, and Wilkeson. When the demand for coal decreased and the supply of the black fuel dwindled, many of the miners and their families left the area. There were some, however, who chose to stay and make these parts their permanent home. These honest, hard working folks infused new skills and traditions into their chosen communities, and it was rumored that one such skill was the art of making some mighty fine moonshine.

I was on my way to Carbonado one summer day to check a steer that was down, and according to the owner, was very weak and couldn't stand. Carbonado was a small community with a population less than 500, located in a heavily forested area near the Mt. Rainier National Forest. The written directions seemed fairly straight forward, but with all the twists and turns on those hinterland roads, it took quite a while to find the place. I finally pulled onto a narrow dirt road that eventually led to an older mobile home that was partially hidden amongst the trees and other vegetation. It looked kinda spooky. This place was really way off the beaten path, there were no vehicles around, no movement,

—— it appeared deserted. Was I at the wrong address? Oh well, I thought I'd better go up there and at least knock on the door. I couldn't hear any movement in response to my initial knocking, — but then the door suddenly opened, and this big, broad shouldered, unshaven, suspender-wearing, brawny fella appeared right before my eyes and said, "Whata ya want?" Looking up at this imposing giant of a man, I asked, "Are you Joe McKay?" "Yup!" He gruffly responded. I told him, "I'm the vet, and I'm here to check out the downed steer you called about." Mr. McKay's facial expressions softened somewhat, but not much, as he said, "Oh yeah, he's out back." I quickly grabbed my medical bags and followed him towards the steer. There he was, — laying in squalor, and looking very pathetic. Upon examination of this poor animal, he appeared thin, weak, extremely pale and anemic, acted as if he couldn't see very well, and had bloody diarrhea. His abdomen heaved as he struggled to breathe. It was a pretty sad situation. Looking around the little pen, I noticed the poor quality of hay that this animal was being fed, and the small adjacent pasture was loaded with bracken ferns. The handwriting was on the wall. "It looks like your steer has bracken fern poisoning, and the outcome doesn't look good at all." I told Mr. McKay. He looked puzzled. "Bracken ferns are poisonous, and when they're eaten by livestock, all kinds of problems can occur, — like tremors, blindness, internal bleeding, anemias, secondary cancers, and sometimes even death." I said. Mr. McKay responded, "Eh,—just put him out of his misery, Doc." So, I did the humane thing, and gave the dying steer an intravenous injection of euthanasia solution and instantly relieved his suffering.

When the job was done, Mr. McKay told me to come inside, and he'd, "pay up". Upon entering the dimly lit mobile home, I was surprised to find three more bruisers sitting there. They all looked rather surly, and stared at me as if I were some kind of intruder. The silence was deafening, and honestly, I was becoming a little uncomfortable. There was tension in the air too, and I didn't feel welcome, — or at least that was my perception. So, in an attempt to break the icy silence, I blurted out with what had to be the dumbest thing I've ever said. — "I hear they make some mighty fine moonshine up in these parts." As I heard those words come rolling out of my mouth, and saw the blank looks on those guy's faces, I thought to myself, "Boy, that was really stupid!" I felt myself sweating, and it seemed like an hour passed before Joe said, "You've never had any good shine before?" "Nope, — never have. —— I've always wanted to try some of the stuff though." I said. Mr. McKay then motioned to one of the bruisers, his son, to go get some "shine". It didn't take long for his son to return with a mason jar filled with what looked like water. Joe unscrewed the lid, poured a small glass half full of the clear stuff, and extended the glass toward me saying, "Here ya go. This here is some really good "white lightnin". — Go slow, now." They all watched as I put the glass to my lips and took my first sip of that high octane concoction. — "HOLY COW! "That stuff is strong, — but smooth." I said gaspingly. My mouth was burnin, and it didn't take long before I couldn't feel my lips. I coughed, and rubbed my now totally numb lips, and that brought welcomed laughs and smiles from all the guys. I thanked them for sharing, and told them that they should be proud of their white lightning, — and I could see how it got its name. They grinned and nodded their heads in approval.

As I was getting back into my truck to leave, Mr. McKay came sauntering up to the cab with a small brown paper bag in his hand. "Here ya go Doc, — a little somethin to take home with ya. — Now, take it easy with this stuff, — it can be habit formin. ——Oh yeah, you don't know where this came from either." He said with a wry grin. I thanked him, shook his hand, and took off. My lips were still numb by the time I got home. —— That really was some mighty fine moonshine.

The Neighborhood Streetwalkers

We lived in a nice older home that was located two blocks from the veterinary clinic. It was a quiet little neighborhood. There wasn't much traffic, and it was relatively safe for dogs to freely roam about. While living at that location, I'd experienced, first-hand, that life can certainly be full of surprises, and sometimes things may not be as they first appear. "Susie" and "Jenny" were clear examples of that.

Susie was a little geriatric Cocker Spaniel cross female who lived on the corner across the street from us. She was a sweet, gentle senior citizen with compromised vision and hearing. Her tongue also constantly dangled out of the left side of her mouth through the space created by some missing teeth. She regularly patrolled the sidewalk, walking at a snail's pace, sniffing the air, and seemingly oblivious to any major sights or sounds, — kind of in her own little world, surveying her domain. She had one very bad habit though, and that was her penchant for sitting smack dab in the middle of the street. There she'd sit, — tongue dangling, squinting her eyes at the cars and giving them the evil eye as they maneuvered around her. It was quite the sight. That was her street, — and she owned it. I told Sandy that little old Susie must have a serious death wish, because one of these days, she could get hit by a car and be seriously injured or even killed. That concerned me, so I kept telling her to get off the street and go home, but to no avail. She just squinted back at me and defiantly ignored my every word. Susie was very independent, stubborn, and wasn't about to move until she felt like it,—so there!

Several weeks had passed, and one day as I looked at Susie, she had that certain "glow" about her. Her tiny tummy was getting a little rounder, and she had more of a swinging waddle to her stride. Could it be? I checked her over, and sure enough, —I felt movement. No doubt about it. This little grandma was pregnant! Susie's owners didn't have a clue as to what she'd been bred to, and didn't seem to care either. Heck, she'd been free to wander the streets, and when one is a street walker, some bad things can happen. I had some legitimate concerns about Susie, because she wasn't a spring chicken, and older dogs can potentially have all kinds of problems with the pregnancy, delivering the puppies, producing enough milk, and even being good mothers. Several more weeks had passed, and then one day, — there she was, — proudly waddling down the sidewalk with four little butterball puppies trailing behind. Susie was so proud of those puppies, and she was a good mom too. She even made sure that the little ones stayed safely out of the street. Wow! What a surprise.

Then there was "Jenny". Jenny was an unkept, undisciplined, hyperactive, grey and white, 8 month old cockapoo. She was a friendly little dog, but a real ditz. Jenny was heavily matted, dirty, smelled, and even though they couldn't be seen, you knew she had to have a pair of eyes somewhere under all that hair. She'd run up and down the sidewalks and streets in hot pursuit of attention from anyone she could find. This hyperactive, frenetic, gyrating little dog would unabashedly jump up on people with her dirty paws, — just trying to play and be noticed.

One Saturday afternoon I noticed a cute, little, well groomed dog leisurely prancing down the sidewalk. "Hey, new people must have moved into the neighborhood, and this nice little poodle cross must belong to them." I said to myself. The little dog seemed friendly, and was actually very well behaved. There was something, however, that seemed a little odd. The "new" dog appeared to be unusually familiar with our street and the surroundings. My lightning fast mind was finally putting all the pieces together. The size, color, and age were about the same, and this little dog with the pink ribbons in her hair didn't really act like a stranger to the area either. Nah, — it couldn't be. Getting bathed, trimmed, and all prettied up shouldn't make that much difference, — should it? I called out, "Jenny?" This "little princess" slowly turned her head toward me with a regal, almost condescending flair, then elegantly trotted off to her house, — or should I say, palace. Jenny had unbelievably become a new person, — er, dog. She had been transformed from a real ditzy ragamuffin into a beautiful princess, and she wanted everyone to know it too. Jenny was now a lady, — with style, and she walked the streets with, —— PIZAZZ!

The Fedora and the Trench Coat

I could tell by the clear blue sky that morning that all was well with the world, and that the coming day was going to be a good one. It was the weekend, the schedule on the books looked fairly light, and we had a day hike on Crystal Mountain planned for Sunday afternoon. I was really looking forward to getting out there and soaking in the beauty and majesty of God's creation.

It was around 10:00 that morning when the clinic phone rang, and there was a very disgruntled lady on the other end of the line. Roberta sat there listening, looked back at me, and rolled her eyes. I always hated that because it usually signaled something rather serious and complicated was going on. Roberta suddenly swirled around in her desk chair, thrusted her arm toward me while tightly gripping the phone in her hand, and with a voice filled with frustration said, "Here,— YOU talk to this lady!" "Hello, Doc Roloff here." I said. The lady took off on a wild tirade. "You vets are all alike! Nobody wants to come out! My cow's got a dead calf in er, and — damn,– now she's gonna die too if she doesn't get some help. Nobody wants to help! —— All that you people want is the money! — You don't care about the animals! You're the fifth one I've called, — everybody says they're too busy and don't have time — nobody is willing to help me,— DAMN IT!!" I had to hold the phone away from my ear because she was yelling and cursing so loudly. "Well, so much for the beautiful day. "I thought to myself. I had to wait for an opening in her diatribe, and when the moment presented itself, I quickly interjected, "Who am I speaking to?" "Gertrude Rempher", she said. "I live over by Federal Way". Oh brother, — that's about 25 miles away, and with her attitude, — no wonder she couldn't find anyone to help her. "Give me directions, Mrs. Rempher, and I'll be right out." I said. "That's MS Rempher, to you — I'm not married." She curtly retorted. I apologized and told her that I'd be out to help her, – in a flash. My ears were still ringing for a while after hanging up the phone. I guess the old saying is true,— "Hell hath no fury like a women scorned." I believed it now, — because I just witnessed it and was on the receiving end too.

I phoned Sandy and asked her if she'd like to go on a farm call over to Federal Way. I explained the dilemma, and told her that I desperately needed her feminine help and moral support on this one, and I'd really appreciate it if she'd come along. Maybe Ms. Rempher would be a little more restrained with a woman present,— maybe not. It'd be worth a try anyway. Thank goodness, — Sandy agreed to go, — and down the road we went. As the verse goes, — "into the valley of death rode the 600".

Amazingly, the directions to Ms. Rempher's place were spot on, and it wasn't long before we pulled into her driveway on the outskirts of Federal Way. Just as I turned off the ignition, this imposing figure, wearing a brown fedora hat, khaki trench coat, and black barn boots materialized next to the white farm house. At first I thought it was a man, but no, — it was Ms. Rempher, and her size matched her booming voice. "You the vet?" She gruffly asked. "Yup, and I'm here to help, — if I can. Where's this cow that's having problems?" I inquired. Ms. Rempher said, "This way.", and off she went. She led us around back of the house to a small red barn, — and there she stood, —a good sized Brown Swiss cow, not looking all that bad or distressed. I started to examine the cow, who's name was "Mabel", and she contentedly chewed her cud throughout the whole ordeal. Next, I had to do a vaginal exam to see if, in fact, there was a dead calf inside, — as Ms. Rempher had expected. As my hand and arm entered the uterus, I felt a small muzzle, and when that little muzzle mouthed my fingers, I instantly knew that we had a LIVE one. I looked over to Sandy, gave her a wry smile, winked, and then cheerfully announced, "We've got a lively little one in here!" Ms. Rempher's face, peering out from beneath the brim of the fedora, underwent a facial expression transformation — from one of extreme skepticism and gloom to downright elation, — in the twinkling of an eye. That hard-nosed doubting Thomas, or Thomasina, actually chuckled and I could see glimpses of a compassionate person hidden deeply in there somewhere under all that stern bravado exterior. She was overjoyed when I managed to free that little LIVE calf from its dark, warm sanctuary. I took a small blade of grass and gently tickled the calf's nostril with it in an effort to make the little guy sneeze. ACHEW! It worked! Snot flew everywhere. A deep breath and loud bellow soon followed. Ms. Rempher was one happy camper and very appreciative too.

Ms. Rempher was a very interesting person, — extremely defensive and distrusting. She'd probably been taken advantage of over the years, and experienced more than her share of rejection and persecution. Her tough talk and rugged attire definitely distanced people, and surely didn't make her a candidate for Miss Congeniality. Anyway, she was happy and smiling now, — seeing that her beloved Mabel was alive, and that she had a beautiful, healthy calf to boot. As they say, "All's well that ends well." Perhaps Sandy and I helped restore Ms. Rempher's trust and confidence in veterinarians, — I sure hoped so.

Our paths with Ms. Gertrude Rempher would never cross again, but the image of that stern, imposing woman, wearing a brown fedora, trench coat, and black barn boots, will be forever etched in my memory. Oh yeah, we did manage to go on that hike up on Crystal Mountain. The sky was clear, the sun was shining, and the view was absolutely breathtaking. The thought crossed my mind, "I wonder if Ms. Rempher has ever seen such beauty? Maybe we should bring her up here sometime, — nah!

The Lumberjack Cook

The timber industry was big business in the Pacific Northwest, and especially in Western Washington. Weyerhaeuser, one of the world's largest wood and paper companies, had its headquarters located not too far from Enumclaw. Weyerhaeuser was a major employer in the area, and directly affected many communities, including Enumclaw. Logging trucks were everywhere, and you needed to watch out for them at all times. They were big, fast, and owned the roads. When passing them on some of those narrow roads, my heart would always beat a little faster, and my palms would become sweaty, because those monsters had a lot of weight behind them, and they were really movin too. Time was money for those drivers, so you'd better get out of their way. —— No problem! It wasn't hard to identify the lumberjacks around town either. They usually wore red suspenders, rugged logging boots, black high water pants, and drove pickups with chainsaws, gas cans, and other logging equipment in the truck beds. The shorter pant legs looked like they'd been in the dryer too long, but there was a reason for them being shorter. It was a safety issue. You see, the shorter pant length made it less likely to get snagged on branches, and also decreased the possibility of the pants getting caught by the chainsaw. Pretty smart! No matter who you met, they often seemed to have ties to, or were affected by the lumber industry in one way or another. Such was the case with Emma Doyle.

It was late in the day, and there weren't anymore appointments scheduled. Great! Maybe I'll get home at a reasonable hour today,

I thought to myself. It would be nice to have dinner with the family for a change. Then the phone rang, and there was that dreaded pause. Roberta wrote down some things, hung up the phone, and chimed out, "You've gotta go out to Emma Doyle's place. She's gotta steer down. It's just outside of town on 264th. You should still make it home on time for dinner." Oh brother, I'd heard that line before, and most of the time, things usually didn't work out that way. Oh well, like the saying goes, "Duty calls and you must attend".

Roberta's directions were right on the money, and it didn't take any time at all to find the place. There it was, an old, two story farmhouse needing paint, hidden amongst an untended windbreak of trees, shrubs, and overgrown, tangled blackberry bushes. I pulled into the short lane and stopped the truck. It looked like a scene taken right out of an Alfred Hitchcock movie, — dark, no movement, and eerily silent. I sat there for a moment, surveying the eerie setting. Suddenly,– a short, portly, mustachioed gent, dressed in a tweed sports coat and Irish driving cap, came sauntering up to the truck. He paused, smiled, and with a sweeping motion of his arm, gestured for me to follow him. It was kind of spooky. I got out of the truck, introduced myself, and wasn't prepared for what happened next. I'd heard people talk fast before,— but not like this guy. When he opened his mouth and spoke — it sounded like a rapid fire, verbal machine gun. I couldn't understand a single word that he said. I repeatedly interrupted him by asking, "What?", but he wasn't fazed, and kept on launching the verbal volleys. Finally, I waved my hands and arms in the air as if surrendering, and pleaded, "Whoa ——SLOWER!" He smiled apologetically,— realizing that he had a communication problem,— he then forced himself to speak slower. His speech was still fast, but now I could understand some of what he said, — at least I got the gist of it. He said, "Come with me to the barn,

— Mother will be coming." I nodded that I understood, and then we were on our way.

We hadn't walked more a few steps when, out of the shadows came a slight framed, petite, elderly, sneaker-wearing dynamo, charging down the steps of the old rickety house. She had her grey hair pulled back in a bun, and together with the black dress, she strangely resembled the farmer's wife in the famous painting entitled, "American Gothic". "I'm Emma," she said. "You must be the vet. — Follow me." So, with long strides and her arms a-swingin, Emma left us in the dust. The little gent looked at me, –raised his eyebrows as he cocked his head, and forced out, "Mutter!"

I got to the barn, and started to examine the steer. He was weak, had pale mucous membranes, and the sclera of his eyes was also whiter than normal. The steer had labored breathing, and was unable to stand. I found thousands of lice and nits (lice eggs), all over his body. They were sucking lice, meaning that they were feeding on the steer's blood. The poor animal was essentially being drained dry, and his chances of surviving weren't good. I placed an IV catheter and started the IV fluids, gave vitamin injections to stimulate red blood cell production, and applied pesticides to get rid of the lice that were robbing the poor creature of its life sustaining blood. I told them that was all that could be done, and we'd just have to hope for the best. I then gathered up all my medical things and Emma's son accompanied me back to the truck. When I opened the door of the truck, there on the seat laid a beautiful hand picked bouquet of flowers. It was Emma's way of thanking me for at least trying to save her steer. That thoughtful act of kindness really touched me. As I was writing up the bill, Emma's son, struggling to talk slower so that I could understand, said to me, "She wants you to come inside for something to eat." I glanced at my watch, and since this was my last call of the day, and I was already late for dinner, I thought that it wouldn't hurt to go inside for a little while. Upon entering the dimly lit house, Emma's son ushered me to the dining room, where a huge, oval, dark oak table was filled to overflowing with wonderful smelling food. It looked like a feast fit for a king, — or a lumberjack crew. It turned out that Emma had been the cook for a local logging crew for many years, and she'd retired only recently. I sat down to eat, and boy did I ever eat!. The food was unbelieveably good, and there was lots of it too. Emma's son, still wearing his tweed sports coat, brought out his favorite Irish beer, and we indulged. It was fantastic! — I was in "hog heaven". Emma didn't say much, she just sat there smiling, simply finding pleasure in having a guest thoroughly enjoying her cooking. I'd become totally stuffed,— to the point where I couldn't eat another bite. I actually had to loosen my belt as I headed out the door to my truck. WOW! — What a meal!

The steer eventually recovered, and Emma made sure to watch out for the lice. I'd learned that those lumber camp cooks could serve up some very tasty food. The only problem was, Emma's recipe books didn't show how to cook for just three people. When I finally got home, I had some explaining to do, because I couldn't eat the dinner that Sandy had prepared, — no room left. Sandy graciously understood, — wrapped up the meal,— put it in the refrigerator, and said with a smile, "That's OK, we'll just have it tomorrow night." —— That was just "hunky-dory" with me.

Why Me?

W e've all had moments in our lives where we've asked the question, — "Why Me?" How do we respond? Alfred Lord Tennyson provided us with an answer in one of his poems. He wrote, "theirs not to reason why, theirs but to do and die". I prefer the vernacular, — "Suck it up, stop the whining, and just do it".

I had many opportunities to apply that philosophy. One such opportunity was being designated the veterinarian on duty at the King County Fair. A veterinarian was needed to examine the incoming livestock, making sure to permit only healthy animals onto the fairground premises. Unfortunately, there were a few over zealous parents who attempted to slip their kid's sick animal into the Fair, Since the animal was sick, it had to be disqualified, denied entry, and sent home. As a consequence, I was called every derogatory name in the book, and even had my ancestry questioned. On top of that, there were several occasions where I was called upon to treat some horses and ponies who were colicy, because they'd been fed pizza and cotton candy by their adolescent owners. It really was a thankless community-service job, and more than once I asked myself the rhetorical question, — "Why Me?".

Charlie Windslow was a master of understatement. It was a day packed with appointments, and time management on farm calls was paramount. Simply put, the day was crazy! I had previously been tipped off to Charlie's antics of slipping stuff in on farm calls, but I had somehow let that bit of info slip my mind. Charlie had initially scheduled six Holstein calves to be castrated. I figured that shouldn't take too long to accomplish, and I'd still stay on my time schedule. When I arrived at Charlie's dairy, instead of 6 calves, as I'd erroneously assumed, he had 40 big Holstein calves, each weighing close to 700 pounds, milling around, needing to be castrated. My first thought was, "Charlie pulled it off again. This will really screw up my time schedule, and now the rest of the day will be a game of "catch up". I really had to hustle! I managed to get the job done pretty fast, and even remembered to save the testicles for Dave Bishop. Dave often asked me to save bull testicles for him because he liked to put on Rocky Mountain Oyster feeds for all of his friends. Trying to be all things to all people wasn't easy, — and once again I asked myself, —— "Why me?"

Now, Dave Bishop was one of a kind. He was a shrewd, wheeler-dealer type businessman, socialite, and self-appointed food critic, who thoroughly enjoyed well prepared food and oddly enough, Rocky Mountain Oysters. On one occasion, he asked me if I'd ever eaten Rocky Mountain Oysters. I told him I hadn't, and probably never would, because the mere thought of eating a bull's testicles was, to say the least, very repulsive to me. Dave said, "Oh Doc, — if they are prepared properly, —they're gooood eating. They taste exactly like regular oysters. I'll bet, — if you ate some, —you wouldn't be able to tell the difference." I told Dave that I'd definitely be able to tell the difference, and surely wouldn't eat any on purpose. Dave just laughed, and said, "Okay Doc, — we'll see".

Several months had passed since I'd last talked to Dave. It was sometime in July when Sandy and I received an invitation to attend a get-together at the Bishop's home, which was located on the outskirts of town. It was to be a casual and relaxed evening of dining and socializing. Dave would be preparing most of the food, and the rest of the menu would be catered. It sounded wonderful and it provided Sandy and me with an opportunity to so something extra special together. It was a fabulous evening, —delicious food, and a chance to meet some very interesting and influential people. Dave made his way through the crowd to personally thank us for coming, and reminded us to sample some of the dishes he'd prepared, — especially the oyster fondue. Sandy and I assured him that we would, and eventually we did try the oyster fondue. — Dave was right. — It was very tasty. Sandy and I thoroughly enjoyed ourselves, and it really was an evening to remember.

On the following Monday, Dave stopped by the clinic and greeted me with, "Doc, glad to see that you and your wife could make it to the dinner. Did you have a good time? The food was great wasn't it." I told him the food was simply outstanding, and thanked him again for inviting us. "How'd you like that fondue, Doc?" He slyly asked. I told him that I'd never eaten oyster fondue before, but it was actually very good. ——"GOTCHA Doc!" Dave said with a big grin on his face. "Those weren't mere oysters, Doc, — they were Rocky Mountain Oysters, — and YOU ate'em, — and thought they were good!" See, I told you that you wouldn't be able to tell the difference." The thought then flashed through my lightning fast mind, — I'd been had! — I'd been set up! —— "Why Me?"

Another opportunity was a palomino gelding named Apache. He needed to be tube wormed, and tube worming wasn't one of my most favorite procedures, — and the horses didn't exactly care for it either. You see, a long rubber tube had to be inserted into the horse's nose, then slowly and carefully passed down into the stomach where the liquid wormer would be placed with the use of a small hand pump. Most horses tolerated the procedure pretty well, but Apache absolutely hated it with a vengeance! He'd rear up and strike out with his front hooves, intending to plant one or both squarely between a person's eyes. He was ultra quick, and had pin-point accuracy too. Believe me, this boy knew what he

71

was doing, — and he had the ability to seriously injure someone. Apache had to be heavily sedated before attempting to pass the tube, and even then, with his head almost touching the ground, and his lips floppy limp, he'd still try to strike with his hooves. Additional hobbles had to be placed on the guy before the procedure could be safely completed. The whole thing turned out to be a real rodeo,— but I got it done. I once again asked myself the proverbial question, —— "Why Me?"

Frank Amsdon was something special. He called the clinic one day, and Roberta answered the telephone. I saw her smile, and while struggling to keep from laughing out loud, she handed me the phone and said, "You really won't believe this. You gotta talk to this man." "Doc Roloff here, what can I do for you?" Mr. Amsdon chimed out, "I've got a bull calf here with 3 testicles, and he needs to be cut." I was, quite honestly, caught off guard, and chuckled as I told him that it would be extremely rare, and highly unlikely for a bull calf to have 3 testicles. I wasn't prepared for his curt response. "Are you new? — Now listen here SONNY, I've been raise'n calves for a lot of years, — and I've probably seen a lot more than you have, — and what I got here is a calf with 3 testicles! —— And I want him cut!" It was glaringly obvious that I shouldn't have chuckled, and I needed to be more diplomatic with this guy, so I told Mr. Amsdon that I'd be right out to check the calf, — and maybe he was right. I made it to Frank Amsdon's place, checked out the calf. Lo and behold, there were only 2 testicles, and there was nothing abnormal. I then gave Mr. Amsdon a short anatomy lesson, showed him the two testicles, and what he thought was a third testicle was actually the scrotum, where the testicles resided. He wasn't totally convinced. He looked at me with a sober expression, and while squinting his eyes he said, "You sure you're not miss'n something?" — I said to myself, — "Why Me?"

A Close Call

The ten o'clock appointment on the schedule simply stated, "dehorn and place nose ring in bull". That didn't sound too tough. I'd done lots of dehorning, but not too many nose ring placements. Those procedures usually aren't that difficult when performed on young calves, but doing them on older and bigger cattle can present a whole new set of challenges. The main concerns with the dehorning procedure are getting adequate anesthesia around the base of the horns to minimize pain, and controlling the bleeding. There usually isn't too much bleeding with younger calves, because the horns are smaller and there's more limited blood supply at that age.

I got the truck stocked with all the medications and supplies I thought were needed for the day's upcoming calls. The schedule said that I'd be going out to Ralph Petre's place for the bull dehorning. I'd never been to his farm before, but Dr. Wagner had mentioned that Ralph had a very upscale hereford operation. I was looking forward to the farm call, and working with some beef cattle again.

It wasn't hard to find the farm because of all the red barns, white corrals, and the herd of white-faced hereford cattle peacefully grazing on the lush pasture. There was no doubt about it, this was the place. I drove up the fence lined lane to one of the the barns where Ralph Petre was patiently waiting. "Mr. Petre, I'm Dr. Roloff, Dr. Wagner's associate. I understand you've got a bull that needs to be dehorned and have a nose ring inserted, right?"

Mr. Petre responded, "Yup, and I've got him tied up in the big barn for ya." I thought to myself, "This is great! He's got the calf all tied up and waiting for me. This should be a piece of cake." We went inside the big red barn, and Ralph nonchalantly said, "There he is". I was dumbstruck! This wasn't a small calf of 100-200 pounds I'd be dealing with. This was a massive, mature hereford bull who weighed at least 2000 pounds, and his HUGE curved horns ominously extended forward and slightly downward from his head. He turned his gigantic, powerful neck and head toward me, stared directly at me, then snorted as if saying, "MAKE MY DAY"! This proud, defiant, and imposing creature could seriously hurt somebody, and that included me. I looked right back at this enormous bruiser, and let him know by my body language that I wasn't about to be intimidated by him. My experience of being raised around beef cattle, and having worked with bulls through-out my youth, had taught me a lot about their body language and how it related to their will and behavior tendencies. This bull was formidable, and I immediately knew that I had to be on my A-game when dealing with him. "Ralph, why are you dehorning this guy now, at this age?" I asked. "Because he's tearing up all the other cattle with those weapons of his. He really knows how to use those things, and I've had enough of it. He's stubborn and he's dangerous too. I need a ring put in his nose so that I can, at least, have some control with him". Ralph said. That was good enough for me. I told Ralph, "Okay, let's do it". He nodded his head in agreement. It was then that I made, what could have been, a fatal mistake. I wrongly assumed that an experienced cattle-man, such as Mr. Petre, would have securely tied and properly restrained such a powerful animal. I'd always reminded myself to never assume anything, but this time, I disobeyed one of my tenets, and that error could have gotten me killed. As I approached the bull to assess the size of the horns, and the amount of local anesthetic I'd need, the bull suddenly whipped his powerful neck, head and curved horns at me with a determined, sweeping motion. There must have been about three feet of slack in the rope, and that extra freedom of movement allowed him to get a good swing at me. His left horn came in toward my abdomen in much the same way that a boxer would throw a hard left hook shot to an opponent's midsection. He connected!!! I flew at least 12 feet across the barn runway, — dazed and stunned by the fact that I had narrowly escaped being gored by the bull. I slowly got back up on my feet and checked to see if I was bleeding or injured, — I wasn't, but the right side of my pelvis was totally numb. The bull's sweeping hook move had allowed the point of his horn to hit me just below the brim of my pelvic bone. I had survived only by the grace of God, because if that horn would have been an inch higher,— it would have passed directly through me, — in one side, and out the other. I would have been completely eviscerated, — and dead! As I regained my senses, I noticed Ralph's face had turned pale, as if he'd just seen a ghost. "You alright?" He asked. I answered, "I think so." Now I started to become perturbed. I pointed my finger at Ralph and told him, "You go tie that guy up really tight this time, — the way he should have been tied in the first place. That's going to be the LAST time that bull's ever going to use those horns on anybody, — and I mean it!" Mr. Petre promptly got the bull's head tightly secured to a support beam. I went up to the bull, looked him eyeball to eyeball, and said to him, "Hey buddy, you remember me? — If you don't, — you will!" I anesthetized the area as best I could, and then proceeded to saw off that bull's weapons. Once that bloody job was finished, I grabbed the nose ring and plunged it through the septum of his nose, making sure that it was firmly in place. Finally, — the ordeal was over. Actually, the whole fiasco was a real adrenalin rush for me, — it was exciting! I guess it was the thrill of dodging a bullet and getting away relatively unscathed, and honesty, I'd be willing to do it all over again. The critical key elements in this situation were, maintaining my self confidence, keeping my composure, not allowing myself to be intimidated, and never showing fear.

I had a very bruised hip and sore pelvis for several weeks, and was thankful to have escaped such a close call. The incident, however, didn't tarnish my fondness of cattle one bit. Heck, I'd grown up on a wheat and cattle ranch, where feeding and caring for the cows was a daily routine. Although I'd been stepped on, kicked, butted, run over, and chased by cattle, I still enjoyed working with and being around them, even if it did involve a close call now and then.

Dale the Chipmunk

O ne of the best things about being a veterinarian in a mixed practice was that no two days were ever alike. It made life very interesting, — and fun. You never knew what kind of animal or medical condition you'd be facing next, and a person had to be mentally prepared for just about anything, — anytime, — day or night. It definitely wasn't boring.

I had just finished performing a spay (ovariohysterectomy) on a cute little cockapoo named Susie, and was in the process of placing her in the recovery room, when Roberta stuck her head around the corner, "Doc, there's someone up front who wants to talk to you." I told her that I'd be right there momentarily. As I entered the waiting room, the man standing by the front counter said, "Hello Doc, I'm Bill Carter from the Weyerhaeuser Company. Do you know anything about chipmunks?" I sure wasn't expecting that type of question, but I told him, "Honestly, — not much!" Mr. Carter smiled and responded, "That's more than I know. You see, we're trying to make a promotional commercial for television that incorporates a chipmunk peeking over a log. The problem is, we can't get the little guy to hold still. He's always moving or tries to escape just as we're about to film. Do you have a sedative or something that would slow him down? — That's what we really need." "My concern", I said, "is that I don't know how a chipmunk would respond to the sedatives I have, and I'd have to estimate a dosage, — that could be tricky. Sometimes those tiny forest creatures can even have adverse reactions to the drugs, and die." "That's okay Doc," Mr. Carter responded. "See what you can do. — I'll tell you what, — I'll leave him here with you for a couple days, — do what you have to do, — and then we'll just go from there. — Okay?" I couldn't believe that I'd agreed to do it, — but I did.

Dr. Wagner noticed me carrying the small cage and its passenger back to the treatment room. He asked, "Hey Doc, — whata ya got there, — some ferocious, rabid, forest creature?" "Nah, a chipmunk that some guy from Weyerhaueser wants sedated for a TV commercial." I replied. "Good luck. That should be interesting." Dr. Wagner responded with a laugh. "Don't kill him." I told Dr. Wagner that I'd do my best not to.

The little guy was cute, and actually pretty good sized for a chipmunk. He was bright eyed, a little on the pudgy side, but still very quick. I managed to find sedative dosages for gerbils and rats, but nothing for chipmunks specifically. Chipmunks weren't all that much different though, — they were all rodents, — so I thought I'd give it a try. Giving a tablet orally to this little speedster was definitely out of the question, so my only option was to administer a subcutaneous injection of the sedative. I calculated the dosage, essentially for a rat, then reduced it by 30%. It took some coercion to get Roberta to assist with giving the injection to "Dale" the chipmunk, but we got it done. Within moments, Dale fell fast asleep. Oops! That dosage won't work for filming. It took a while for him to sleep it off, so later in the day I adjusted the dosage and tried again. This time it worked, — sort of. Dale got pretty drowsy and his little eyes got squinty, but now he could be easily handled. I propped him up on a rolled up towel that substituted for a log, and he didn't move. — He sat there as if he'd just 'tied one on". His little head gradually sunk down and his eyelids began to close, but when I snapped my fingers, his head came back up and his eyes were wide open, — for a few seconds, then they slowly closed again. — VOILA!!! This dosage should work!

Bill Carter showed up at the clinic the following day, as he said he would. I explained what I'd come up with for a workable sedative dosage, and the timing of the finger snap to get the eyes to open for filming. I gave little "Dale" the chipmunk his happy shot, then off he went with Mr. Carter. I never heard back from Mr. Carter about how things worked out. I thought the commercial had probably been scrapped for one reason or another. Anyway, it had been a fun case. Then, about a month later, while Sandy and I were watching television one Sunday afternoon, a Weyerhaeuser commercial appeared on the TV. At the end of the commercial, there was a short clip of a little chipmunk peering over a small log. It was "Dale"! I knew it was him, because I'd recognize those squinty little eyes anywhere. I said to Sandy, "Hey look at that. I helped make "Dale" a TV star.

Unbelievable

It was late summer, the days were longer, and the sun didn't set until about 8:00 p.m. It had been a good day, pretty routine, and I was even getting home at a decent hour. Time to pull out the ole barbeque and grill some of that fresh salmon I was given by a client earlier in the day. I was really looking forward to spending some quality time with Sandy and our young son, Eric. Veterinary medicine can definitely cut into family time, and a person needs to take advantage of every opportunity that comes their way.

The barbecued salmon was, without a doubt, outstanding! We were having fun and thoroughly enjoying the evening together – until the dreaded phone rang at 7:30 p.m. Sandy answered the phone and handed the receiver to me. I listened to the concerned individual on the other end of the line and said, "I'll be right out. Put some pressure on it until I get there."

Sandy asked, "What is it?"

"A horse got shot with a rifle, right through the front leg," I said. At least we had a little time together as a family and a fantastic BBQ salmon dinner to boot.

On the drive to the farm, I pondered over how the horse got shot, especially at this time of day, at dusk. It didn't take long to get to Mr. Hume's farm, and it was obvious that I'd found the right place because there was a rather large group of people standing around a horse, and one of the guys was holding a rifle. Something really weird was going on here. I got out of the truck and promptly went over to the horse to examine its injuries. He was a Morgan

81

gelding, a smaller-statured breed of horse, and was quietly stand-ing there, acting very nonchalant about the whole incident. There was no active bleeding, just some passive blood trickling down the back of his right front leg. The bullet had passed completely and cleanly through the flexor muscles located between his knee and chest, miraculously missing the radius bone and any of the major arteries, veins, and nerves. This horse was, without a doubt, totally graced out! I cleaned, medicated, and bandaged the wound and also started him on antibiotic therapy.

I then told Mr. Hume, "I'll be back in a couple of days to re-check the horse. You know, -your horse was really very lucky. He literally dodged a bullet." That comment brought a few chuckles and helped lighten the atmosphere a bit. Well, the show was over, and most of the onlookers took off. The fella I'd seen with the gun turned out to be Mr. Hume, and he confessed that he'd accidently shot his own horse. I looked him straight in the eyes and asked, "How in the world could you ever do that? What were you shoot-ing at? A bear, a coyote, or what?"

He sheepishly looked down at the ground and shook his head no. He then looked up and said, "You may not believe it, but I was trying to scare off a Bigfoot with a shot, but I hit the horse by mistake. Can you keep a secret and never tell anyone about this place? I don't want people running all over my property looking for Bigfoot."

I assured Mr. Hume that I wouldn't tell anyone. I wasn't pre-pared for his next question, "Doc, do you believe in Bigfoot?" The look in his eyes left no doubt whatsoever that this man had indeed seen a Bigfoot, or some creature that resembled one. I replied, "Honestly, I have no basis for making a judgment either way."

"When you come out to check the horse in a couple of days, Doc, I want to show you something, and then you can decide for yourself if you believe or not," he said.

I'd scheduled the recheck on the horse for Saturday afternoon because I had the afternoon off, and there'd be more time to spend with Mr. Hume. His property was located adjacent to the Mount Rainier National Forest, a huge forested area. If there was such a creature as Bigfoot, and if he did roam this area, he'd have ample cover to go undetected. I still secretly had my doubts, but I kept an open mind.

Mr. Hume had the horse waiting for me when I arrived at his farm. The wound was healing nicely and no longer required bandaging. Mr. Hume was pleased and relieved because he was fond of that horse and felt awful about the shooting incident.

He then began to share with me his experiences involving Bigfoot. He'd owned the property for only five years, but the previous owners told him many stories about Bigfoot encounters. One of the stories was extremely interesting. The previous owner was an eighty-eight-year-old woman. She told Mr. Human that as a child, she played with her big hair friend many times. Her friend would come to her bedroom window at night, she'd slip out the window, and they'd play together in the small orchard nearby. The elderly woman always spoke fondly of her big hair friend.

I asked Mr. Hume if he'd ever seen a Bigfoot or Bigfoot tracks. He said he'd found footprints and bedding areas. He'd sent hair and fecal sample to research facilities for analysis, and the results come back: species unknown! I asked Mr. Hume if he could show me where he had found a Bigfoot footprint. He was more than willing to oblige.

We then proceeded to the edge of the pasture that abutted the Mount Rainier National Forest, climbed over the fence, and entered a heavily wooded area. There was heavy undergrowth and a nearby low area where water had collected, making the ground soft and moist. As I was parting some of the grass to expose the earth, there it was, a huge footprint! We also found a resting area, an impression of where the creature laid down, and some hair that really smelled foul. Suddenly, I had this overwhelming sensation that we were being watched. The hair on the back of my neck began to stand up, and I froze. I slowly turned my head toward Mr. Hume, who was about twenty feet to my left. He was also motionless and had an alarmed expression on his face. He then slowly motioned with his head that we'd better leave. We slowly and carefully withdrew from the area, and then Mr. Hume said to me, "Did you feel that? – We were being watched by something." I told Mr. Hume, "I felt it too – That was really weird!" Was it Bigfoot? I don't really know.

That was an incident that I'll never forget! Two men, simultaneously sensing imposing danger, the finding of a very large footprint, about fourteen inches long, under some pressed down grass, and collecting some very unusual looking, and stinky hair. I'd become less of a Bigfoot skeptic. Some people may think Bigfoot is a hoax, but I know what I saw and the feelings I'd experienced. I've held true to my word as well. I've never divulged the exact location of that unbelievable encounter.

Good Timing

We've all experienced serendipitous moments in our lives, especially when things unexpectedly worked out to our benefit. Sometimes those spontaneous moments of good fortune can even rescue us from difficult and unfavorable circumstances. A case in point, the outcome of one particular call.

Clayton Zuker was a conscientious cattleman, and his registered Hereford operation exemplified that fact. He was very attentive to the health and welfare needs of his cattle, so it was not surprising that he quickly detected a problem with one of his prized bulls. The bull had been favoring his right front leg for several days and Mr. Zuker suspected that the bull had somehow sprained its leg. When the limping got worse and traces of blood appeared where the bull had been walking, it was time to call the vet. Lucky me!

It was that season of the year when the sun didn't shine. If the sun did peek out, you'd wonder what you did wrong. Day in and day out, the sky was cloudy, rain fell almost constantly, ranging from light drizzles to heavy downpours. Some peopled called it liquid sunshine, but that was certainly a matter of opinion. The flip side to all of the moisture was the beautiful scenery of lush pastures, dense green forests, and all the rivers and streams. It was a good trade off, at least that's the way I rationalized it. One thing for sure, rain clickers and rubber boots were very much in vogue, and the standard attire of the day.

Mr. Zuker had the bull secured in the squeeze chute when I arrived. The bull's hooves were encased in mud, so it needed to be thoroughly washed off before the problem could be assessed. Once the hooves were clean, the source of all the limping stuck out like a sore thumb. There, deep in the web of the cloven hoof, was a bloody, firm, tumorous mass, about two inches in diameter and it was forcing the digits of the hoof to spread wider apart than normal. The growth was an interdigital fibroma, and sometimes they're loosely referred to as bovine corns. That type of fibroma tended to be firmly attached, grew around and entrapped arteries and veins, which in turn resulted in making the surgical removal of the mass a rather difficult, time-consuming, and very bloody procedure. I knew what I was up against, but there were no other options. The tumorous mass had to be surgically removed.

The two-thousand-pound bull had to be immobilized in order to eliminate pain and constant leg movement during the operation. The absolute last thing I needed was to have a two-thousand-pound patient thrashing his legs all over the place during surgery. We found a suitable soft, grassy area where the bull could be safely laid down, and then I proceeded with the anesthesia. So far, so good. Just as I was preparing the surgical site, a few raindrops began to hit my slicker, but I continued in spite of the drizzling rain. As I'd expected, the fibrotic mass was firmly attached and had grown extensively around the blood vessels in that area. Unfortunately, many of the arteries and veins had to be severed in order for the mass to be completely removed, and that resulted in substantial bleeding. Blood quickly filled the surgical field and obscured my view of the arteries and veins that desperately needed to be located and ligated (tied off) to stop the hemorrhaging. A tourniquet and gauze sponges were totally ineffective. Then suddenly, as if an answer from above, the rain increased from a slight drizzle to a heavy downpour. The intensity of the rain flushed the blood from the incision site, and made the severed arteries and veins clearly visible. They could now be easily identified, clamped, and ligated. Man, was that perfect timing or what! Now I could see what I was doing, and it didn't take long after that to successfully remove the fibrous mass. I bandaged the hoof, the bull woke up, and the ordeal was over.

Thank you, Lord, for the rain! That downpour of rain came at the right time, and was a true blessing. It really was a serendipitous moment.

A Day in the Life

It has been said that, "variety is the spice of life". If that saying is true, and in most cases it is, then the life of a veterinarian is very well seasoned.

The first order of business each day was to take a look at the appointment book, see what was on the schedule for the day, and get mentally prepared for the onslaught. The schedule always looked so organized and manageable, — on paper, but we all knew that after the first appointment, things would invariably change, and the rest of the day would be a wild ride, — but it was still fun. The reality was that the term, "typical day" didn't exist in our vocabulary.

The day began with well-check exams and vaccinations on two cats, and a dog named Skippy. They were all healthy except for the occasional fast moving little brown guy, scurrying in, around, and through the hair, attempting to make its great escape. — Fleas! Fleas were a common finding in that part of the country, and the pesky, little, annoying opportunists were a relatively easy problem to deal with, except when they jumped off the animal and got on you. The patients were vaccinated, treated for fleas, given snacks for being good, and were then good to go. Now on to the next case.

I was scheduled to vaccinate two calves just a couple of miles south of town. These calves needed to be vaccinated against bacterial and viral diarrhea, rhinotracheitis and parainfluenza virus of the respiratory system, and pinkeye, a type of conjunctivitis of the eye. They also needed to be wormed against internal parasites, and checked for lice. Once that was completed, and I was about to leave for my next scheduled appointment, Mr. Ensor, the owner, came running up to the truck. "My wife wants to know if you could take our dog,"Lucy", back to the clinic with you — check her over — and I think she needs some vaccinations too. We'll come in later in the afternoon and pick her up." I asked," Sure, what kind of dog is she?" Mr. Ensor replied, "A doberman, but she's nice,— she just looks mean. She rides well, and she should be good with you." I thought to myself, ——SHOULD —— be good! What happens if she – ISN'T – good with me in the in the truck? Then, Mr. Ensor hollered, – "LUCY". Bounding around the corner of the house came a big red doberman with head held high and ears raised in full alert position. Mr. Ensor managed to grab her by the collar, got her attention, looked sternly into her eyes and commanded her, "Lucy, now you BE NICE to this man!" Oh joy! Now he's telling her to be — nice—. The thought flashed through my brain, "What have I gotten myself into?" Mr. Ensor then opened the passenger door and ordered, —"IN". Lucy hesitated at first, but with the second command, up and in she jumped, and promptly situated herself as close to me as she could possibly get. I swear, we must have looked like we were joined at the hip. As I drove down the road back to town, any oncoming driver probably couldn't tell who was actually driving the truck, me or Lucy. In fact, she had nudged so close that I asked her several times, "Lucy, do you want to drive?" We made it back to town, and I stopped by the grocery store to pick up a can of pop, and when I came out of the store, there she sat, smack dab behind the steering wheel. This big, mean-looking dog, head up and ears alert, appeared to be guarding my truck. People gave my truck plenty of room. No one was going to get close to that truck except me. As I got into the truck, Lucy acted like I was her long lost friend who she hadn't seen in years. She yipped and licked my hands and face in sheer delight. Lucy may have looked tough, but she was a real cream puff. From that day on, red dobies and the name Lucy would always produce fond memories. I dropped Lucy off at the clinic, and was off again to the next case, an EMERGENCY, a horse with a stick through its ear.

As I pulled into Virginia Cumming's pasture, I could see several people standing with a a sorrel quarter horse, whose name turned out to be "Buck". Buck appeared to be mildly agitated, and intermittently flicked his left ear in an attempt to dislodge the 1 inch x 12 inch wooden stick that had impaled the lower part of his ear. Each time Buck flicked his ear, the stick moved past his eye, causing him to react by jerking his head in an effort to avoid being hit by the the object. That only made things worse, because he'd now become very head shy. I quickly grabbed a towel and placed it over Buck's eyes in an attempt to calm him down. It worked! Now to assess the situation. The stick couldn't be pulled through, instead, it had to be cut close to the ear, and removed in two pieces. The procedure was fast, effective, and with minimal bleeding. The only problem was that the one inch puncture hole left by the stick, near the base of the ear, didn't lend itself well for closure with sutures (stitches). It would heal fine as an open wound. Buck now had a permanent identification mark,— er hole. A real topic of conversation. A couple antibiotic injections were given, and — on to the next case.

The last farm call of the day was to Bill Talbert's place. Bill was an ex-professional football player. He'd gotten out of pro-football for some reason or other, bought himself a small ranch, and settled into semi-country life. He didn't have much acreage, but enough for a couple cows and a pig named, "Clarissa". Mr. Talbert was physically a very big man and he'd most likely been a tough interior lineman in his glory days of pro-football, but Clarissa had stolen his heart. He met me at the truck when I pulled into the driveway, and proceeded to emotionally explain that Clarissa had injured her eye, and now she was in severe pain and unable to open her eye at all. I told Mr. Talbert, "Let's take a look, where is she?" Mr. Talbert said, "out back". I grabbed my medical bags, and we were on our way. What I saw next was definitely not what I had expected to see. Mr. Talbert had led me to an extra large doghouse with the hind end of a pig sticking out of the doorway. "There she is, the poor girl. Please do something to help her." He pleaded. My first thought was, I've got to get her out of there in order to examine her eye, but all of Bill's coaxing hadn't budged her an inch. Every time he touched her she grunted defiantly, and then Mr. Talbert stopped. I suggested that maybe we could pull Clarissa out far enough so I'd be able to check her. — NOPE!! Each time we'd attempt to grab ahold of her legs, she'd scream bloody murder, and the thought of dismantling the doghouse wasn't an option to Mr. Talbert. I noticed that there was a small space on her right side, and thought that maybe I'd have enough room to slide in beside her, and with a small flashlight, I might be able to check out her eye. Vet school hadn't prepared me for this maneuver. Anyhow, there I was, wedged between a pig and the doghouse, in ultra-tight quarters, attempting to examine a pig's eye. If she attempted to bite me, I had nowhere to go. Heck, I could barely move, let alone get out of her way. Somehow, I managed to apply a local anesthetic to her eye, and once the pain was gone, she opened her eye, and it could finally be examined. The cornea of the eye was swollen, edematous, cloudy, and ulcerated. Corneal ulcers can be very painful and are extremely sensitive to light. No wonder she was holding her eyelids shut and in so much pain! During the eye exam, I found a piece of barbed plant material wedged between the lower eyelid and the eyeball itself. That was the problem, — that was the culprit! It was a cheatgrass awn, sometimes called a foxtail, it scratched her cornea, it hurt , and Lucy was rubbing her eye in an attempt to get the thing out. Unfortunately, there was more harm done than good. I removed the cheatgrass awn, medicated the eye, and began my Houdini moves in an attempt to dislodge myself from the confines of that doghouse. When I finally emerged, and showed Mr. Talbert what I'd removed from Clarissa's eye, he was so overwhelmed with relief and appreciation, that he actually started to cry tears of joy. That man really did love his pig. All's well that ends well.

The day had finally come to an end. Time to go home and have a beer. — After that day, I really needed and deserved one. I was tired, but happy, knowing I'd helped some animals and their owners as well. A good night's rest was really needed, because the next day was guaranteed to be more of the same, — but I loved it!

OUT ON MY OWN

A New Beginning

Owning my own veterinary clinic somewhere in Eastern Washington had always been my ultimate goal. While attending a veterinary conference in Seattle, I'd heard that the area in and around Four Lakes, near Spokane, was ideal for and in need of a veterinarian. So, Sandy and I decided to take a weekend excursion to Eastern Washington and check it out. As we approached Spokane on Highway 2, I took an errant turn onto Brooks Road, which led us directly to a charming little town with a lake actually located within the city limits. The town had a very unique and interesting history that involved the healing properties of the lake water, so that's how it got its name, —Medical Lake. We drove around and explored the little City of Medical Lake, liked what we saw, and thought that this quiet little town definitely had possibilities! Sandy and I both felt that this was a good place for us to risk it all and step out on our own. Now, the town of Four Lakes was just 5 miles further down the road, but fate had stepped in, and we never did make it to our original destination.

We knew that it would be a bitter-sweet relocation process for us. The decision to leave Enumclaw was very difficult because we'd made many new friends, and thoroughly enjoyed the beautiful surroundings with Mt. Rainier nearby. I also greatly appreciated the opportunity to practice veterinary medicine with Dr. Wagner, and I'd learned a lot from him, but I had that unquenchable desire to pursue my dream of someday owning and operating my own veterinary practice. It was a huge step of faith,— but Medical Lake would eventually become our new home, and the place where I'd hang my veterinary shingle for many years to come.

It's been said that, "beauty is in the eye of the beholder". When we saw an unsightly, abandoned service station, littered with vintage posters and smelly empty oil cans, located in the center of the city of Medical Lake, we thought that it had the potential to be resurrected as a new veterinary clinic. It was, without a doubt, truly a diamond in the rough, — real rough! Not only would we be removing a perennial eyesore from city center, but we'd be providing a new business to the community. A win-win situation that would come to be enthusiastically welcomed by the townspeople. A future client, Mel Holmes, handcrafted and donated a large wooden veterinary sign as a welcome gift. He'd painstakingly chiseled out the letters MEDICAL LAKE VETERINARY CLINIC into two massive timbers, and JAMES A ROLOFF DVM into another massive timber. Then he proudly mounted them onto the front of the building. It looked great!

Word of a new veterinarian in town spread like wildfire throughout the community and the surrounding area. The renovation project had not yet been completed, but that didn't stop people from coming to our residence, seeking veterinary services for their pets. Necessity truly is the mother of invention, so I modified our little used RV into a make-shift mobile veterinary clinic, and it sufficed for the time being. Sandy and I had scheduled an open house for the clinic on a Sunday afternoon in October. It was intended as a time to meet and greet the townspeople of Medical Lake, but it didn't turn out that way at all. You see, many people seized the opportunity to get long overdue veterinary care for their four footed family members. I finished seeing patients at 9:00 that evening. We were tired, but happy with our new home town and its friendly people. It really was a new beginning and a dream come true.

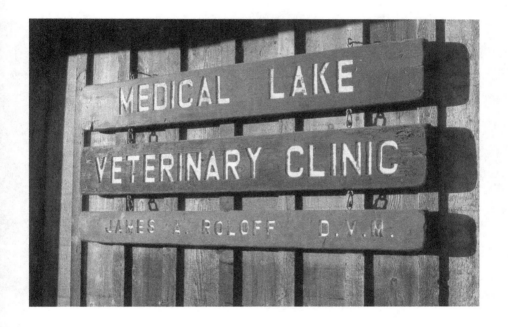

Brutus

Dogs are often referred to as, "man's best friend", and rightly so. Dogs tend to be loyal and faithful companions who shower us with sincere devotion and unconditional love. As a general rule, they view their people as consummate masters and providers. However, there are always exceptions to the rule, and Brutus was a prime example of a dog who didn't get the memo.

Brutus, a stout Norwegian Elkhound, was an independent, self-serving guy who operated outside the box. He considered himself the center of the universe, and all of life revolved around him. In addition, he had a checkered history of unabashedly expressing his disdain for veterinarians and veterinary hospitals. His owners alerted me to that fact before he arrived at the clinic. I cautiously introduced myself to Brutus, and proceeded to examine him. It didn't take long to see that Brutus had a serious problem. He was unable to urinate, and the urinary bladder had become extremely distended, causing him to experience intense pain and discomfort. X-rays revealed a urolith (bladder stone) lodged behind the os penis structure, totally occluding the urethrae and preventing the passage of urine. That resulted in the over distention of the bladder. Death could result if this condition were to go untreated. Brutus had experienced a similar problem previously, but the urolith was smaller and passed successfully, but not this time. The urolith was too large and it would be impossible to pass without surgical intervention. I immediately performed an emergency surgery, called a urethrostomy, removed the offending urolith, and reconstructed a new permanent opening for Brutus so that he'd never have the problem again. The delicate surgery was successful, and Brutus was then placed in a nice warm recovery cage where he'd slowly wake up from his slumber. When he awoke, he was much more comfortable, the intense pain was gone, he was in a nice warm place, and to him, — life was good again.

From that moment on, in Brutus' mind, that was HIS feel-good cage, and I was his good buddy. He actually liked coming to the clinic after that day. He'd barge through the door of the clinic and make a beeline to the recovery room where he'd check out HIS special cage. He'd give it a few sniffs, making sure that all was well and that it was still there. It was to be an expected routine with Brutus that would be repeated many times for years to come. Oh yeah, he never experienced another blockage after that surgery was performed.

A Kitten Named Arrow

S ome idioms are strangely true. "A miss is as good as a mile", "close but no cigar", and "stranger than fiction", are three idioms that perfectly describe the case of a very lucky kitten.

A young boy burst through the front door of the clinic with a calico kitten cradled in his arms. He exclaimed with panic in his voice, "I found this kitten by my house.— Somebody shot it with an arrow. — Can you do something to help it?" The kitten, about 4 months old with big green eyes, was resting nonchalantly in the boy's arms, — and there was an arrow lodged in its face and sticking out the other side of its back. I'd never seen anything like that before. The kitten didn't appear to be overly distressed except for when she attempted to move her head. It was then that the shaft of the arrow wiggled slightly, and it greatly impeded her lateral head movement. The kitten's vital signs appeared to be normal, there was no active bleeding, and her lungs sounded clear and normal. She was understandably somewhat apprehensive, but who wouldn't be with an arrow lodged in their face. The kitten needed to be placed under anesthesia and the situation evaluated before attempting the removal of the arrow. The point of entry of the arrow was on the left side of the kitten's face, near the corner of her mouth. It bounced off her cheek bone and exited by the back of her jaw. It then reentered by her left shoulder, passed between the vertical processes of her thoracic vertebrae, and exited on her right side. This sweet little kitten had been literally skewered by an arrow, and in the process, all the major arteries, veins, and nerves had been missed. It was basically a miracle! The wooden shaft of the arrow needed to be cut in order for it to be removed. I then cleaned, medicated, and sutured (stitched) the traumatized entry and exit holes. We were done. The kitten awoke from the anesthesia uneventfully, and moved her head around in all directions as if nothing had happened. It was pure joy, watching her jump and play like a normal kitten again, especially so soon after surgery.

As it turned out, the kitten was a nameless stray without a home. I wasn't going to let that continue, so I named her, "ARROW", gave her all the necessary vaccinations, and found her a home where she would be safe and loved. Arrow's case really did turn out to be, "stranger than fiction".

Tempting Fate

One of my mother's favorite sayings was, "Haste makes waste". I should have been a better listener, because on one particular occasion, my overconfident haste almost resulted in me getting permanently wasted.

A cow with a sore on her tail was my first farm call of the day. It was a short 5 mile drive to Frank Slind's place. Frank was essentially a hobby rancher with limited acreage, and a herd of three Shorthorn-cross cows. Mr. Slind wasn't much of a talker,— actually, he was a very quiet, reserved man. So, when asked where the cow was located, he simply pointed out in the direction of the small pasture. There, standing quietly and tied to a lone tree, was a compact roan-colored cow, rhythmically swishing her tail. I asked Frank, "Do you have a squeeze chute or something where we could restrain her movement?" He curtly responded, "Nope". Well, that answered that! Wow, this case was going to be more difficult to treat than I thought.

The swollen, bloody, foul smelling sore was located high up at the base of her tail, and her feeble tail swishes weren't effective at keeping the annoying flies away. As I approached the cow to check out the sore, she instinctively knew that something was up, and began frantically pivoting around the tree in a vain attempt to escape. This case had become a real challenge, and was getting dicier by the second. The cow was now in survival panic mode, and her constant movement made it nearly impossible to give her a tranquilizer injection. I was running out of ideas, — but then I remembered a seldom used "barrel-roll" rope restraint technique. The rope would be tied around the cow's neck, then maneuvered round her shoulders and flank, and when pulled it would apply pressure to the nerves, which in turn would slow the cow's movements and also prevent her from kicking. That seemed like a good plan! Just as I was getting the rope prepared, a big black fly suddenly landed on the cow's right ear. Instantly, and with lightning-fast speed, she kicked off the fly with her hind hoof. It was a blur of motion! Boy, was she good, — ultra fast and accurate too! That was a wakeup call for me to be very cautious. I carefully proceeded to tie the rope around her neck, then placed the rope over her back. The next step was to reach under her belly and grasp the dangling end of the rope and pull it towards me. Hindsight is always 20/20, and suggests that I should have used a stick or broom handle or something to reach the rope, but I was in too much of a hurry. Knowing full well that the cow had a very fast kick, I nevertheless thought I was faster. I mistakenly thought that I could quickly grab the rope, and move my head out of the way before she would kick. WRONG! The moment I reached under her belly, — POW! She caught me flush on my left jaw with a right hook, or should I say a right hind hoof. I'll never forget the sound of the impact inside my head. It sounded like a baseball bat hitting a telephone pole. My eyeglasses flew about 12 feet, and my head must have spun around because I later found hoof scrapes on my right shoulder. The amazing thing was that I was still standing after getting nailed by that powerful knockout blow. I saw a few twinkling stars, and my ears were ringing, but she didn't knock me out! I took a lickin' but kept on tickin'. After regaining my senses and composure, I went at it again, only more carefully this time, and completed the rope restraint. I was then able to successfully clean, treat, and medicate the sore on the tail.

It goes without saying that I was very fortunate and truly graced out. I could have been seriously injured by tempting fate with my overconfident haste. I'd learned my lesson the hard way, — and as usual — Mother knew best!

Double Trouble

The odds of lightning striking twice in the same place are, quite honestly, slim to none. Likewise, the odds of saving a client's two animals from near death conditions is also pretty remote. However, sometimes things just happen to work out in a way that totally defies the odds. Such was the case with a cat named "Hoss" and the family cow.

Phone calls to the vet clinic usually involved the scheduling of appointments, animal care questions, or salespeople pitching something or other. Then there were the emergency calls, — they'd really get the juices flowing. Like the time when our receptionist hung up the phone and chimed out, "A lady just called, and she's on her way in with a cat that just got caught in the fan belt of her car." A statement like that would always conjure up all sorts of macabre-like mental images. When cats tangle with fan belts, — cats never win! Severe and often life threatening injuries invariably result. A bonafide emergency case was on its way, staff members knew what to do, and immediately began preparations for the cat's arrival.

It wasn't long until Christine Anderson stormed through the clinic door with a large, brown tabby farm cat named "Hoss", draped over her bloodstained arms. Hoss had sustained some major injuries from getting caught in the fan belt. — He was really messed up and in serious trouble. There were lacerations on his head, ears, legs, and back, plus severe bruising around his left eye. But the worst injury was to his abdomen. The skin from his ribcage to his groin had been torn away, exposing the detached abdominal muscles along the ventral midline. His intestines and other internal organs could be clearly seen moving beneath a tissue-thin structure called the peritoneum which lines the abdominal cavity. That extremely thin, delicate, transparent structure was the only thing preventing total evisceration (disembowelment) from taking place. Hoss was also in a state of shock, and his chances of surviving didn't look good. Intravenous catheters were immediately placed, and medications were given to counter shock. Once Hoss was stabilized, I turned to Christine and tried to explain that animals with injuries as severe and extensive as Hoss's usually didn't survive, but she didn't seem to grasp what I was saying. Instead, she stood there very composed, and calmly said, "Oh Doc, — I believe in you, — you'll save him." I thought to myself, "How can she be so sure? She's either in a total state of denial or doesn't understand what's going on here." Anyway, I told her that I'd do my best to put Hoss back together, — but I couldn't make any promises. She just smiled, — and seemed to understand THAT!

Hoss was carefully placed under a general anesthetic, and we got the show on the road. It was a team effort involving me and the veterinary assistants, — shaving, cleaning, debridement, medicating and the actual surgical reconstruction. Rebuilding that little guy was a long, painstaking procedure. Hoss had a strong will to live, —everything went well, and he made it through the surgery with flying colors. Granted, he looked a little Frankensteinish, with stitches everywhere on his body, but his mucous membrane color and respirations were good. As I placed him gently into the recovery cage, I told him, "Hoss, little buddy, you did good. You hung in there and made it through, — this time. Now, stay away from those fan belts, because I don't want us to keep meeting this way, — Okay!

Christine brought Hoss back to the clinic several weeks later for a recheck. He'd made a remarkable recovery, and looked almost as good as new! I told Christine that when I first saw Hoss's torn and beat-up little body, I didn't think he'd make it. I really had my doubts. He'd beaten the odds, but it cost him 8 1/2 of his 9 lives lives to do it. He was, plain and simple, lucky to be alive. Christine smiled and said, "Doc, I never doubted for a moment that you could save him." I thought to myself, "At least one of us did."

It was later that year when Christine again called the clinic with another doozie of a problem. It didn't involve Hoss this time, thank goodness. Hoss was just fine, but her cow wasn't. She explained, "I think my cow has a dead calf inside of her. She's been out there in the pasture for several days, not moving much, and really stinks! I don't know how long she's been trying to have that calf, — but I think she needs some help." I told Christine that cases like that never ever turn out good. A cow with a dead calf inside for an extended period of time, usually results in the cow becoming toxic, septicemic, and in most cases, the cow dies. It's not a pretty picture! Sometimes it's more humane to put the cow out of her misery instead of letting her continue to suffer. Christine responded, "Doc, I know it's a long shot, but could you at least take a look at her, and see? Maybe you could help her like you helped Hoss." I couldn't believe what I was hearing. I said, "Christine, you don't understand. There's a 99.999% chance that this cow of yours is going to die from the advanced septicemia." She responded by saying, "That's okay, Doc. I have confidence in you, because you saved Hoss and he was almost a goner." I told myself, "Oh brother, — just go out there and check the cow out. She'll probably be dead by the time I get there."

It was a 20 mile drive to Christine's place, and she was waiting by the out buildings when I arrived. As I was getting out of the truck, Christine asked, "Can you smell that?" The nauseating stench of rotting flesh permeated the air. — It was BAD! "Where is she?" I asked. Christine pointed towards the open pasture. Way out there in the distance laid a black, white-face (Hereford-Angus cross) cow. "That's her." Christine said. I had a bad feeling about this one, especially when you could smell her this far away. Someone once told me that a good way to counter foul odors was to place some Vicks Vaporub in your nose. I always carried a small jar of the stuff in the truck for moments like this, — and believe me, — NOW was the moment to give it a try! Pack those nostrils FULL!! So, with trusty Vicks stuffed up my nose and my stout rubber, shoulder-length, obstetric gloves on, I proceeded to examine the cow. Her mucous membranes were pale and tacky to the touch, and her respirations were weak and shallow. This poor gal was septic, dehydrated, and in big trouble. — Not a good sign! As I inserted my arm into the pelvic inlet and uterus, it felt abnormally warm, — actually hot, due to the infection, inflammation and decomposition of the dead calf that was taking place inside of her. The rotten stench was almost overpowering, — even with all that Vicks up my nose. I felt a hoof, grasped ahold of it, and as I began to position it into the pelvic inlet, it pulled loose. It was one of the dead calf's legs, and when I pulled it out, — it looked bad. The hair was falling off, and the muscles tissue looked pale and resembled boiled chicken, — only worse. It stunk to high heaven too! Christine surveyed the scene and said, "It looks really bad, doesn't it." I told her, "If this cow lives, it will be a miracle. Downer cows with dead, rotting, decomposing calves inside, rarely survive. — They die!" I continued to remove the dead calf, one decomposed piece at a time until, — finally, — the entire corpse was removed, and laying on a stinking pile. I then flushed out the uterus with disinfectants, instilled antibiotics, and gave her a couple potent antibiotic injections. I told Christine that

I was going to attempt to get the cow to stand up, but cautioned her not to expect much, because the cow was so weak and septic. I then knee'd the cow in the hindquarters and simultaneously hollered, "Come on, get up!" — No response. I knee'd her a second time, and this time she staggered to her feet, — a little wobbly, but she was standing and looking around. UNBELIEVABLE! A few moments later she sauntered off a short distance, and started to eat grass! Christine started to laugh, cheer, and clap her hands, — all at the same time. I just stood there smiling, amazed, and speechless. "You did it again, Doc. You did it again!" Christine said while smiling ear to ear.

That cow had defied the odds too. She steadily improved, and yes, she lived. The rotten stench had penetrated the rubber gloves and had gotten into the pores of my skin. I washed my hands and arms with everything imaginable, but to no avail. It took several weeks to wear off, and during that time, I was referred to as "Stinky Doc" at the clinic. Looking back, lightning did strike twice in the same place for Christine. Hoss and her cow were "LIVING" proof.

Baby Huey

The original Baby Huey was a lovable cartoon character . He was a large, clumsy, goofy baby duck in diapers. The Baby Huey I knew as a patient fit the description perfectly, except for one minor detail, instead of being a baby duck in diapers, he was a huge, happy-go-lucky Great Dane.

I'll never forget the first time I met Baby Huey. He was scheduled for a routine physical exam and vaccinations, and his grand entrance into the clinic was an event not easily forgotten. This enormous fawn colored Great Dane, weighing in excess of 200 pounds, came bounding through the door, knocking over tables and chairs, with his owner flailing on the end of the leash like a lure on the end of a fishing line. The expression, "Bull in a china closet", was appropriate in his case, except that Baby Huey had more of a Ferdinand type personality. He was a very friendly, clumsy goof, who loved everything and everybody — Happy, Happy, Happy, — Oh boy, Oh boy, — Can I sit on your lap? — type of guy. He really was a fun patient, and could easily cheer up someone's day, if he didn't bowl them over first. Physically, he looked more like a small horse than a dog. He had a huge head, long legs, and enormous paws that resembled ping-pong paddles. Baby Huey was, without question, one super sized hunk of love, very appropriately named, and a real kick in the pants!

Several months later the owner called the clinic and frantically told our receptionist, "My dog just ran in front of the hay mower and got his legs cut real bad. Is Doc gonna be there?" It was Baby Huey, and it didn't sound good! When Baby Huey arrived at the clinic, he was unable to stand, let alone walk. He was placed on a stretcher, and four people struggled to carry him into the clinic, where he was immediately transferred to the surgery table. Pressure bandages had been placed around his left front and left rear paws in an effort to slow the hemorrhaging, but they were now totally soaked with blood. The bleeding had to be stopped soon or Baby Huey could die from loss of blood. He was quickly sedated and anesthetized, the blood-soaked towels were removed, and the spurting arteries were located, clamped, and ligated (tied off). Once the bleeding was under control, the extent of tissue damage could then be more easily seen. There were severe lacerations just above the paws, in the metacarpal area of the left front leg, and the metatarsal area of the left hind leg. The rapid back-and-forth motion of the hay mower's sharp sickle blade had made two very deep transverse lacerations, about four inches apart, on both of his legs, — cutting arteries, veins, tendons, and nerves. It was a MESS! Four tendons on each leg had been severed in two places, — making a total of 16 separate tendon cuts. One would have been bad enough, — but 16! The four inch pieces of severed tendon had shifted from their original positions, and that further complicated the situation. The nightmare would be trying to figure out where each piece had to go, and it essentially resulted in comparing the sizes of the severed ends.

Tendons are notorious for being slow to heal, and sometimes they don't heal properly. Without adequate tendon support, Baby Huey might never be able to stand, let alone walk or run. His odds of recovery were not good at all, and his owner knew it. They were devastated, and even considered putting Baby Huey down. — I didn't want to see that happen. It's been said that necessity is the mother of invention, and I had an idea that might help Baby Huey. I told the owners that perhaps using a non-absorbable permanent suture to reattach the tendons might work. Baby Huey's tendons were pretty good sized, the sutures could be anchored more securely, and would have a better chance of holding. I also told them that I'd never performed a surgery like that before, — I'd be essentially "venturing outside the box", so to speak, but if everything went right, then Baby Huey might, — just MIGHT, have at least a chance of walking again someday. I couldn't make any promises, but making an effort to help him would be far better than putting him down. The owners, with tears in their eyes, didn't hesitate for a moment before they chimed out, "LET'S GO FOR IT!"

Baby Huey was immediately taken to surgery, and the reconstruction process turned out to be a very intricate, tedious, and painstakingly slow procedure. Finding the displaced severed tendons, properly matching them up to their respective ends, and delicately reuniting each one, was repeated sixteen times. Closing the skin lacerations was the final step. When the surgery was completed, I was totally spent, — both physically and mentally. I was confident that the tendons had been properly reattached, and was hopeful that the sutures would hold. — Time would tell.

Baby Huey spent the next several weeks under house arrest, with his left front and rear paws heavily bandaged in an attempt to restrict movement at the surgical sites. The "happy" pain pills also helped relieve some of the discomfort and slowed him down somewhat too, but he was still a handful for his owners. When he began moving his paws, that was an encouraging sign, but when he walked several steps, his owners were absolutely elated! The sutures held, Baby Huey eventually was able to run, and he became his ole clumsy, lovable self again.

The procedure was a long shot, — it probably shouldn't have worked, but it did. Baby Huey was one of the most challenging and rewarding cases of my veterinary career. I'm thankful that I went "outside the box" with an idea, and it worked to save a friend's life.

Imprinting

Zoological imprinting is defined as a behavioral condition wherein a young animal can come to recognize another animal, person, or thing as a parent or object of habitual trust. "Bugsy", a little six week old buff-colored cocker spaniel puppy was a prime example.

A man stepped up to the reception counter, plopped down a small puppy, and said, "Something's wrong with this pup. He doesn't look right, and the mom keeps pushing him away. He's the runt, and he doesn't get around like the other pups. I don't have the time to mess around with him, so I want you to just put him down." Melanie, our receptionist, ushered Mr. Torkel and his puppy into the exam room. As I started to examine the tiny puppy, Mr. Torkel said, "I don't want him examined,— just put him down!". I looked Mr. Torkel straight in the eyes and told him, "I won't do that without examining him first. Mr. Torkel, the ONLY reason I'll ever consider euthanasia is to relieve the pain and suffering of an animal who is incapacitated or terminally ill, — for humane reasons, not for convenience." Mr. Torkel responded, "Well, forget it then, I'll take him somewhere else and have it done." Somebody else might, but not me. I felt that this little guy at least deserved a chance at life, so I said to Mr. Torkel, "I'll tell you what, Mr. Torkel, you sign ownership of this pup over to me, and then he'll be mine. I can then give him a fighting chance on my dime, and it won't cost you a cent." Mr. Torkel thought for a second, but no more than that, and said, "DONE!" He turned around, walked out of the clinic, and I never saw or heard from that man ever again.

I was now the proud owner of a malnourished little runt of a dog who just happened to be a hydrocephalic with an enlarged head and protruding eyes. He was, without question, sitting squarely behind the 8 ball. I gently placed the little guy into the pocket of my light blue smock, patted him delicately, and told him, "Little Buddy, now that you're mine, let's see what we can do for ya." I walked out front and showed the staff my new little pocket pet. "Whatcha gona name em, now that he's yours?" Melanie asked. I looked down at the little bulgy-eyed puppy in my pocket, and said, — BUGSY, that's what I'm going to name him. Yeah —— "Bugsy" —— because his eyes kinda bug out in a cute sorta way."

Bugsy was definitely exhibiting the signs associated with a hydrocephalic case. Hydrocephalus is a condition where there is excess fluid in and around the brain, causing the eyes to bulge and the head to become more dome shaped. The bones of the skull are softer and more flexible at this age, because the fontanels (junction spaces) between these bones haven't yet ossified(hardened) and become fused. So, the excess internal fluid puts pressure on these bones and causes them to spread somewhat, and that makes the head look bigger. Sometimes the fluid absorbs and the condition resolves, sometimes it doesn't, which could then result in seizures and possibly even death of the individual. Shunts were not a treatment option in Bugsy's case. His condition was not as severe as some, so there were possibilities that the problem might normalize with "tincture of time".

Over the next few weeks Bugsy spent a lot of time riding in my smock pocket. I guess you could say that he was my sidekick. The bulginess of his eyes seemed to be resolving somewhat, he was eating well, more playful, and becoming a pretty spoiled little guy too. No doubt about it, Bugsy was improving, and it was also becoming increasingly apparent that he thought I was his "MOM".

It was around that time frame that one of our clients, named "Vi", had lost her old Cocker Spaniel to cancer. She'd visited the clinic several times, saw Bugsy, and was totally smitten with him. I noticed how Vi's eyes would light up with joy when she saw the little guy, and there was definitely a mutual attraction between those two. I'd come to the realization that I wouldn't be able to carry Bugsy around in my pocket forever, and that he needed a home where he'd be loved and cared for 24/7. Vi lived only three blocks from the clinic, so I'd be able to see him quite often. That was important to me, because I'd become very fond of Bugsy as well. Vi and Bugsy seemed to be made for each other, and it was beginning to look more and more like a match made in heaven.

As time passed, Bugsy's medical condition totally resolved, and he'd become very handsome and healthy. He was one happy camper! Every time Vi took Bugsy for a walk, and passed by the clinic, he'd pull on the leash towards the door, wanting to come in to visit. Vi often laughingly said, "I have this dog at my house who I feed and care for, but you know what,— he's not really my dog,— he's yours! He thinks you're his MOM. He'll always feel that way, — but I still love him.— I can deal with that." I smiled, gave Vi a big hug and said to her, "That's what's called imprinting, Vi. Bugsy's a doubly blessed boy, because he's got something that most dogs don't have, — TWO MOMS."

"Bugsy", my pocket pet

"Bugsy", all grown up, happy and healthy

The Unexpected

Ray Winston and his wife, Vivian, lived on a small ranch located a few miles south of town. They enjoyed country life, and of course accumulated an assortment of farm animals.

Vivian had become interested in showing dogs, and selected a Pekinese male from a very reputable breeder, hoping that someday he'd eventually become a champion. The dog had a pedigree name that was a mile long, but they just called him, "Howdy". He had the ideal looks and outstanding lineage, but unfortunately not the mindset. Howdy thought he was a herding dog, like a Blue Heeler cattle dog, but somehow got morphed into a Pekinese body. He just loved to get out there, down and dirty, and to him, the barnyard was his show ring. His favorite sport was herding the cows, and without a doubt, he was fearless. At times he'd come dangerously close to being kicked but his low profile served him well. As the cows kicked in response to Howdy's annoying heel biting, their hooves sailed harmlessly over his little head. He was quick for such a short-legged little guy, and usually, his timing was spot on.

Overconfidence can often lead to disaster, and one can go to the well just so many times before coming up empty. Such was the scenario with Howdy. Vivian called the clinic one day with a voice beset with dreaded concern, and relayed to the receptionist that she was on her way to the clinic with Howdy, because his eye had been badly injured. Vivian didn't exactly know what happened, but she had a good Idea. After examining the type of injury and the extent of tissue trauma, it was obvious that Howdy hadn't ducked fast enough, and a cow's hoof connected squarely with his left eye. There was considerable damage. Unfortunately, Howdy's left eye was prolapsed (moved forward and downward) out of the socket, and the optic nerve had been severed. Regrettably, Howdy's eye could not be saved.

I will forever be amazed at the will and resolve of some animals. We could all learn some valuable lessons from them. Howdy was undaunted with the loss of his eye. To him, having just one eye was nothing more than a minor inconvenience. The possibility of him ever entering the show ring had evaporated, but his love of life hadn't diminished one iota. He was the same happy-go-lucky, fun loving, barnyard dog, but now he was sporting a permanent wink. He didn't stop herding cows, but he did learn from his mistake. Howdy now had a very healthy respect for a cow's kick, and from that time on, he gave the cows a wider berth and made sure to duck a little faster.

"Howdy"

Assuming

One of the meanings of the word, assume, is to suppose something to be the case without proof. Sometimes assuming can be advantageous, but on the other hand, incorrect assumptions can result in a bucketload of regrettable consequences.

Ron Winston called the clinic and told our receptionist that he had a pig that needed to be castrated. No problem! Most male pigs are altered at a reasonably young age, and since Mr. Winston didn't specify the age, it was assumed that he was referring to a younger animal. Such procedures are relatively quick and easily performed on the young ones.

Upon arrival at the Winston place, Ron told me that the pig was caught up in the barn. I appreciated that because now we wouldn't have to go through the "greased pig chase" routine. I grabbed my equipment and together we headed to the barn. Once inside, and seeing the "pig" that I was supposed to castrate, — my facial expression must have resembled the "dead fish" look, —— mouth gaping and eyes opened wide. This wasn't a 30 pound pig! Standing right there before me was a 500+ pound Landrace boar, with testicles the size of eggplants, and he didn't appear too keen about the idea of being transformed into a eunuch. There were no stanchions around to help confine him, so Mr. Winston came up with the brilliant idea of putting a rope around the boar's neck and tying him to the massive 3 inch thick wooden cow manger. I had my reservations about doing that, but there weren't many options, — in fact none! This huge boar was not about to have his testicles removed without anesthesia. The proven technique for sedating a large boar was to inject the anesthetic into one of the testicles. As the boar began to absorb the drug and proceeded to fall asleep, the injected testicle would be removed first, and there would be ample time to remove the remaining testicle before the pig woke up. That all sounded quite reasonable. I asked Mr. Winston if he was ready and he said, "let's do it".

I calculated the anesthetic dosage and prepared the syringe. I then grabbed ahold of one of the enormous testicles, and at the very moment he felt the initial touch of the needle, he let out an ear-splitting, bellowing squeal that could have been heard in the next county. He jerked his powerful, muscular neck with tremendous force and instantly dismantled the hay manger. Once free from restraint, he then started running around the enclosure with a huge 3 x 12 inch x 10 foot wooden manger plank dangling from his neck. This whole affair was rapidly turning into a real fiasco. The huge boar wouldn't let us get close enough to even untie the rope, and who could blame him. He kept running and squealing until finally he got his big head stuck into the opening of a large metal farrowing crate that was situated in one of the corners of the barn. That farrowing crate (a structure that protected the piglets from being rolled upon when the sow was farrowing/giving birth) was heavy, but the boar easily lifted that crate onto his shoulders. He continued his evasive maneuvers, and now he was not only dragging a large wooden plank, but he was toting a farrowing crate on his back as well. Suddenly, as if by an act of providence, the crate got wedged into a corner. My moment of opportunity had presented itself, and I quickly took advantage of it. I raced in there and performed the castration so fast that he didn't really feel or know what was happening. DONE! Eventually he managed to back out of the farrowing crate, and the squealing stopped.

WHEW!!!! Mission accomplished, and best of all, no one got hurt. That whole incident was a very valuable lesson for me. In the future, I would make every possible effort to NEVER again ASSUME anything.

Mikey

There once was a television commercial that featured a cute little boy who liked to eat just about anything, and his name was Mikey. The tag line of the commercial was, "Mikey likes it". Those three simple words epitomized one of my closest friends.

Joyce Beauchet was a different sort of person. She was a single, self-proclaimed successful businesswoman from Southern California who moved to the Pacific Northwest to seek anonymity and isolation. She chose not to have a telephone, and was emphatic about keeping her personal matters totally private. Ms. Beauchet simply did not want anyone to know who or where she was. In addition, she chose to conduct all business transactions by cash only, thereby leaving no trail of financial activity. One might say that she was a person who raised many eyebrows, and who was, without a doubt, a very eccentric individual who better not be double crossed.

It was one of those high intensity days at the veterinary clinic, and time management was a priority. I had just finished an appointment, when the receptionist interjected, "Doc, there's a lady on the phone who is very unhappy. She says that someone dropped off a cat at her place, and she doesn't want it. She'll have someone shoot it if you don't take it." I couldn't let that happen so I told Janice, "Just tell her to drop the cat off with us and we'll find it a good home." I thought to myself, "Not another one!"

About an hour later, Joyce Beauchet made her grand entrance and unabashedly plopped a young cat, around 16 weeks old, on the front counter, then sternly said, "Here, it's yours!" She turned around, without even a thank you, and abruptly departed. Left behind and sitting calmly on the counter, was perhaps one of the most beautiful cats I'd ever seen. He was a red Classic Tabby. The color pattern of a Classic Tabby is quite unique because of the bull's-eye marking pattern symmetrically located on the sides of it's body. This young cat was very striking to look at, and instantly made himself at home in his new surroundings. Actually, he seemed relieved, and who could blame him. As I picked him up, an infectious purr-motor instantly erupted and continued as he gently nestled into my arms. I was smitten with the little guy, and knew, right then and there, that he'd found a new home,—— with me. I'd always wanted a red cat, and knew that someday, if I ever found the right one, I'd name him, "Mikey". Well, that someday had come, I'd found him, thanks to Ms. Beauchet, and this little guy's name would, most definitely, be Mikey.

It didn't take Mikey very long at all to settle in as the resident mascot of the clinic. He conveniently situated himself on the office counter, and became the clinic's official greeter and PR (personal relations) cat. He was good at it too, and it wasn't long before he had his very own fan club. Adults and kids would often come into the clinic just to get their "Mikey Fix". He really grooved on all the petting and attention, and truthfully, he'd come to expect it. He didn't discriminate either, in fact, he'd didn't care if a person liked or disliked cats, he'd still befriend them. We'd often hear some anti-cat people say, "I usually don't like cats, but this one is different. — I like this one! What's his name again?" I'd say, "Mikey or Mike whichever you prefer. You know why he's different? He doesn't think he's just a cat, he thinks he's a "Purr-son"." That statement probably wasn't too far from the truth.

Mikey had a unique ability to sense a person's loss, and would suddenly appear and offer his consoling presence to them in their time of need. Over the years he provided needed comfort to many. He truly was very special and one of a kind. On other occasions, whenever anyone talked to him, he'd vocalize to them in varied tones and inflections as if having a friendly, meaningful conversation. It was amazing to see.

Mikey was a blessing to me in many ways, and he was by my side through thick and thin. He lived a long and happy life, and will be fondly remembered by all who knew and loved him. I will forever be grateful to Ms. Beauchet for complaining about that dumped off "cat", because she provided me with a devoted friend and confidant who greatly enriched my life.

"Mikey"

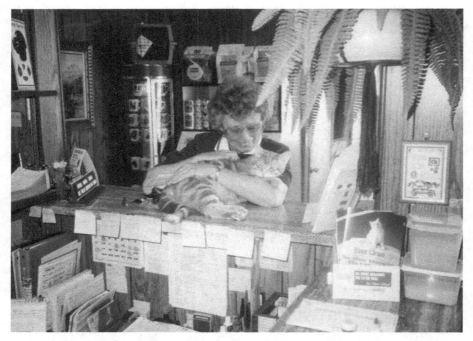

Cybil getting her "Mikey Fix"

Once in a Lifetime

Almost everyone is familiar with the publication, "Ripley's Believe It Or Not", and knows that it focuses on the bizarre and unusual. It can be quite fascinating and interesting to read some of that stuff. So, it shouldn't come as much of a surprise to us when we encounter something very unusual and rare, because certain things in life really are stranger than fiction.

Mr. George Cravits called the clinic that beautiful Spring morning with the startling news that his cow had just given birth to a two-headed calf, and it was still alive! I'd studied about and seen pictures of cases like that in vet school, but I'd never seen an actual, LIVE, two-headed calf up close and personal before. I was really looking forward to seeing this one. So, I grabbed my medical bags and equipment and was on the road in a flash.

A two-headed calf is an extremely rare occurrence. Most are delivered dead, or if born alive, they don't survive very long. It's also very unusual for a cow to deliver a two-headed calf without veterinary assistance, because the head size is often too large to pass through the birth canal. In that case, a caesarean section or an episiotomy would usually be necessary to deliver such a deformed calf. However, in Mr. Cravits' cow's case, she delivered the deformed calf without any complications, and that in itself was totally amazing.

I arrived at the Cravits ranch within minutes and quickly made my way to the calf. I found Mr. Cravits kneeling next to the recumbent Hereford calf, supporting the calf's head in his hands.

"Have you ever seen anything like this before, Doc?" He said. "No, never have, not even in vet school. I'd only seen photos, but never the real thing." I responded. The calf was definitely alive and breathing. One of the two centrally located eyes slowly blinked. The calf had two distinct muzzles, two lateral eyes, two central eyes, two ears, and the heads were fused/joined in the middle. The calf attempted to move his head/heads, but was unable to raise them because of the increased weight. The little guy opened his left muzzle slightly and made a feeble attempt to bellow, but there was no sound. The ultimate outcome was glaringly obvious, — this calf wasn't going to survive. I thought to myself, "The vet school should really have a chance to see this calf before it dies." I told Mr. Cravits, "This calf needs to be transported to the Washington State University Veterinary School right away. It's about 90 miles from here, — and the vet school would really appreciate it, and could learn a lot from this little guy." Mr. Cravits generously complied, and I immediately loaded the calf into my truck, and down the road we went. The little calf, as expected, lived only two days. He was unable to stand, nor could he eat. He was humanely put down, but provided the veterinary school and students with a wealth of valuable information, — so he didn't die in vain.

Two-headed calves are a very rare birth, and in most instances, make widespread, if not global, news. This little guy was no exception. There was extensive local and regional television and newspaper coverage, and he was written about in various veterinary journals as well.

I'd found the saying to be true. Some things in life really are stranger than fiction. I know. I was there, and it was a once-in-a-lifetime experience.

A Match Made in Heaven

Golden Retrievers have the reputation of being gentle, fun-loving dogs, who seem to just go with the flow and have that c'est la vie attitude about life. That's probably why they are such a popular breed.

I first met Delicia, a two year old spayed female Golden Retriever, when her owner, Steve Thorten, brought her to the clinic because he was concerned about some recent changes in her behavior and activity. She used to play fetch with the ball and liked to go for walks, but she'd lost her enthusiasm for all that, and now just moped around. Mr. Thorten went on to say that due to his busy work schedule, and not being home very much, he was afraid that she'd just lay around and get fat. "Mr. Thorten", I asked, "How long has Delicia been acting this way?" "Quite a while." He anwered. When I asked Mr. Thorten if there had been any recent changes in the household, he thought for a moment and then said, "Yeah, — I guess. The cat used to keep her pretty busy, and they played together almost constantly, but the cat got hit by a car and died." — BINGO! I told Mr. Thorton "I think Delicia has been grieving, because she's lost her little friend. What we need to do is is try to find her another companion, preferably a cat. Maybe that would solve the problem.

Several days had passed, and as I was pulling into my drive-way after a busy day at the clinic, a little red-orange colored, tabby kitten came trotting over to the car. It held it's tail up high in the air, and seemed quite friendly. I looked down at that scrawny little kitten and said, "Hi there little buddy,— what's your name?" Just then, my neighbor, Bill, came walking around the corner of his house. "Hey Bill, what's your new cat's name?" I asked. "Oh, that thing isn't mine. It's been hangin around here the last couple days. Somebody must've dumped him off." Bill responded. All the while this little rag-a-muffin was prancing around with its tail in the air and he kept rubbing up against my pant legs, marking me as HIS new possession. He looked up at me as if to say, "Hey you, — don't you know I'm yours? Boy, — are YOU lucky — or what!" As I picked up the scrawny little stray, I immediately saw fleas scurrying and weaving through his hair like downhill skiers traversing a slalom course. The little guy's ears were also filled with dry crusty debris, suggestive of ear mites, he had a nasal discharge, weepy eyes, and then on top of it all, he sneezed directly into my face. Yet, as bad as he looked, he kept purring and kneading away with his paws. This kitten was a mess, but a happy mess, and he needed a lot of help. So, I placed this little vagabond into a carrying crate, and off to the clinic we went for an "extreme makeover". He got a bath, had his ears cleaned and medicated, was treated for fleas, vaccinated, wormed, and had his eyes cleaned too. He'd gotten the "Full Monty", and didn't complain at all. He was one little happy camper, now that he'd been all cleaned up. Life was good, or at least a heck of a lot better. Now, — he needed a name. The most striking feature about this kitten was his red-orange colored hair coat. We decided to name him, "Rudy", because one of the meanings for the word rudy is,— red hair or skin. It seemed to be a good fit for him.

The next task at hand was to find Rudy a good home. Delicia came to mind almost immediately, but the question was, would they get along. I called Mr. Thorten and told him that we might have a little friend for Delicia, and he was receptive to the idea. He knew how much Delicia missed the other cat, and was hoping this kitten might get her out of the doldrums. Mr. Thorten picked up Rudy within the hour, and now, time would tell if it was the right move.

Several days later I received a phone call from a very ecstatic Steve Thorten. He said, "Doc, you won't believe this, but those two hit it off the moment I let the cat out of the crate! They acted like long lost buddies, and they're even sleeping together. Delicia has been licking and grooming him so much that he's covered with slobber and is wet most of the time, but he doesn't seem to mind. Thanks Doc!" I told Steve, "It seems like a match made in heaven, doesn't it." He wholeheartedly agreed.

Delicia and Rudy —— what a wonderful success story. Delicia regained her zest for life, and Rudy found a loving home. It couldn't get much better than that! Those two became devoted companions to each other, and remained inseparable for many many years.

"Rudy" & "Delicia", friends forever.

The Unsinkable Molly

Margaret Tobin was a survivor of the ill fated passenger ship, Titanic. It was reputed that she rowed lifeboat #6 for seven and one half hours and delivered herself and her fellow passengers to safety. She was the only woman to do such a thing, and that act of courage, will, and stamina earned her the nickname, "The Unsinkable Molly Brown".

I once had a patient whose name was Molly, and she too displayed tremendous courage, a strong will, and unequaled stamina in overcoming a potentially devastating injury. She was a 3 year old Brittany Spaniel with true grit, and was without a doubt, the canine version of the famous, "Unsinkable Molly Brown". Molly was a very gentle, affectionate, 30 pound Brittany Spaniel, who had boundless energy and loved to hunt. She was a pleasure to have as a patient, because she was easy to work with and always seemed eager to please. I really liked that little girl.

It was late September when Roger Carney, Molly's owner, called the clinic to set up a time to have her leg checked. As Molly entered through the front door of the clinic, it was glaringly obvious that she'd sustained a major injury to her right front leg. She was carrying (holding up) the leg, and when she attempted to place the paw, it knuckled over at the carpus. The leg was unable to support any body weight whatsoever. Molly was ushered into the exam room, and I began an assessment of her condition. Her leg was severely swollen, edematous, the dorsum (top) of the paw and foreleg were badly scraped and bloody, and there was no response to pain stimulation of the paw. In addition, the righting reflex (paw placement) was absent. I couldn't detect any broken bones on palpation, and x-rays confirmed that fact. It didn't look very promising. At that point, all findings indicated a radial nerve paralysis, and that type of injury could be either transient (temporary) or permanent, depending upon the degree of damage to the nerve. If permanent, she'd never be able to use that leg again. I asked Mr. Carney if he knew what happened and when the injury occurred. He looked down towards the floor, paused momentarily, and with a tone of regret in his voice he said, "I accidentally hit her with the pickup a couple weeks ago, but I thought she might snap out of it." The scrapes on the paw and foreleg appeared to be the result of a more recent injury, so I asked him if he knew what may have caused those injuries. He said that he'd taken her out hunting, and the scrapes were from her dragging the leg through the weeds and underbrush. — That was unbelievable! Molly still had the will to hunt, — using three legs and dragging the paralyzed one. I told Mr. Carney, "I'm sorry, but her leg doesn't look good at all, and with the nerve paralysis, I'd recommend that the leg be amputated for her welfare. If we don't, she'll continue to drag that paw, it will then become severely infected, and could eventually be life threatening. Mr. Carney said that he'd think about it, but for now he only wanted to treat her with antibiotics and ointment for the scrapes. He'd erroneously convinced himself that if the leg were amputated, then she wouldn't be able to hunt. I assured him that Molly would still be a better hunter on 3 legs than most dogs are on all four, but he still declined. My hands were tied, and I honestly felt sorry for Molly.

Two weeks had passed, and Mr. Carney brought Molly back to the clinic. Her leg was now severely infected, and she had become septic. Molly was gravely ill, and her life was definitely in peril. There was no other option at this point —— amputate the leg or put her down. Finally Mr. Carney realized the gravity of the situation, and signed the consent form to amputate the leg. We were good to go! I patted Molly on the head and said to her, "Molly, hang in there with me, we're going to get you through this, and then you'll be able to hunt again. — Okay?"

We got Molly all hooked up to the IV fluids, and prepped for surgery. It was a lengthy procedure. I amputated the leg high, at shoulder level, and reconstructed a protective cushion of muscle over the remaining portion of bone. The leg, along with all the devitalized necrotic tissue, was successfully amputated. Antibiotics and pain meds were administered, — and it wasn't long before she started to wake up. Molly was a great patient! What a trooper! When she was discharged the next morning, she was raring to go, and already appeared to be feeling much, much better! Everybody got excited as we watched Molly come hop-running down the hallway. Even Mr. Carney smiled, — now with some signs of hope and optimism in his eyes.

A week had passed, and it was time to recheck Molly. I saw Mr. Carney pull up with his pickup in front of the clinic. When he opened the door, Molly jumped out and took off running down the street. She ran faster on three legs than most dogs could on four. When Mr. Carney finally caught her, he was the one who was winded. Molly looked and acted great! Everything was healing well, and in another couple weeks she could once again be out there hunting. Needless to say, Mr. Carney was very pleased and thankful.

Molly had overcome extreme adversity with courage, and a very strong will. She continued to be an outstanding hunting dog, and proved to everyone that she was indeed, —— the UNSINKABLE Molly!

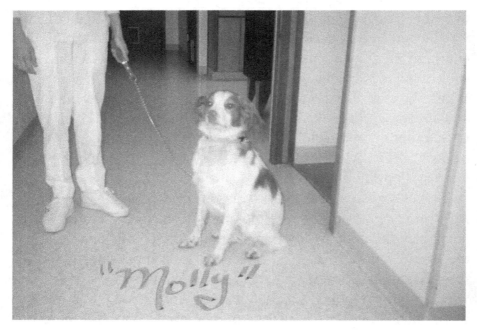

"Molly" with all four.

The Three Amigos

Good intentions are what they are,— plans put into action with hopes of positive outcomes. As we all know, our good intentions don't always result in the manifestation of what we purposed. It has even been said that the road to hell is paved with good intentions. So, if that be true, it becomes very apparent that many good intentions go unfulfilled. The question then is, — how do we respond?

Sandy's grandmother, Kate, lived in a nice retirement center that had a small aviary placed in the center of the main lobby. When we visited her, we'd pass by the large birdcage that housed around twenty small birds of varying colors, ranging from grey and white with red on their heads to simply brown and white. They all appeared quieter than most birds, and their soft chirping was very soothing to the soul. That pleasurable sound seemed to have a calming and almost hypnotic effect to it. I told Sandy, "What do you think about getting a bird like that and placing it in our waiting room? I think the clients would like that. Don't you?" Sandy agreed, and I guess you could say that our intentions were good.

We went to a pet store and described to the clerk the type of bird that we wanted to buy. She told us that the bird we were looking for was called a Zebra Finch, but she had just recently sold the last one. She did, however know of a bird breeder and wholesaler who had lots of them. So, off we went in hot pursuit . When we found the place and entered the building, the loud incessant noise created by all the squawking, chirping and whistling was enough to drive a sane person mad. I wondered, how in the world could anyone work in such a noisy place like this. It wasn't long before a fella noticed our presence, waved acknowledgement, and approached us. I noticed that he moved his hands up to his ears and was fiddling with something. He was adjusting his hearing aids! This guy was either deaf or very hard of hearing, and that's why all the racket didn't bother him, —— he tuned it out! Smart! He then ushered us into the main room, which was much quieter, and asked us what kind of bird we were looking for. I told him that we wanted to buy a Zebra Finch. He asked, "Just one?" He then went on to say, "You shouldn't have just one. You'll need two or more so that the birds don't get lonely." I reluctantly went along with his recommendation, but specified only two males because I wasn't interested in the hassle of raising birds. He then told me that having just two males wasn't a good idea either, because one of them is usually more dominant, and would likely pick on the other one, and then there'd be problems. He recommended that we purchase three. Wow, how could such a simple idea get so complicated? I finally gave in, and the guy caught up three nicely colored male finches. In the end, we walked out of there with three male Zebra Finches, a large birdcage, two designer perches, and a big bag of special finch food. My initial intent was to get one little soft-chirping bird at minimal cost, but here I was, walking out of the place with a mini aviary, and a major investment.

Once the birds were all set up in the waiting room, it didn't take long to realize that dogs and cats rushing up to the birdcage wasn't a good idea. So, all the paraphernalia was moved into my office, and the three birds seemed to like that much better. Mikey, the clinic cat, would get right up next to and on top of the birdcage, but they didn't seem to be bothered by him, in fact, they sorta liked him. Initially the birds got along together pretty well, so we called them, "The Three Amigos". Well, all that was about to change too. One of the birds was becoming more dominate and started harassing and pecking on the other two. Not good! I ended up purchasing another birdcage just for him. That rowdy little mouthy guy was becoming a pain! I started calling him, "PITA", because he had become a real — Pain — In — The — A_ _. The other two needed names too, so we named them, "Shazbot" and "Tookus". Those two were good boys and both made those soothing chirps that we'd hoped to hear, but Pita remained his obnoxious self, and continued to disturb the other two. I had no other choice but to get Pita out of there, which meant eventually taking him home.

It took a while, but Sandy and I became pretty fond of ole "Pita". We placed his cage in a room where he could see all the outside bird action, and that really made his day! Any sharp sound, in the house, on the radio or television would set him off. He'd start his mouthy chattering. When you would go up to his cage and ask him how he was doing, he'd charge right up to you, ruffle up his feathers, and chew you out. This cheeky little bird definitely did not fit the Zebra Finch mold, but he was alot of fun. He was a great escape artist too. Many times I had to play, "catch the flying finch mid-air". On one occasion, Sandy forgot to secure the cage door, and when she didn't hear Pita sounding off as usual, she went in to check. The cage was empty and no Pita in sight. Sandy looked down, and sitting quietly right beside her desk was "Bob", our bobtailed cat, and there were finch tail feathers sticking out of his mouth. Sandy gently grabbed ahold of the tail feathers and sternly commanded, "Bob, open your mouth!" He slowly opened his mouth and Sandy pulled out a LIVE, but wet Pita, totally unharmed. Sandy quickly put him into his cage. He sat for a moment, shook his feathers back into place, then proceeded to chew everybody out again. What a schmuck! We loved him anyway.

The average lifespan of a Zebra Finch is said to be around 5 years. Pita lived to be 15 years old, and that was truly amazing. He was exceptional in so many ways, and lived life to the fullest, for a Zebra Finch. Pita was a real kick in the pants, and although he was a cheeky little fella, he'll always be fondly remembered as a, "Good Amigo".

The "Three Amigos" & Mikey

Code Blue

Color codes are designated to various emergency situations encountered in medical facilities. Code red indicates a fire emergency, code orange refers to a hazardous material spill, but a code blue signals a medical emergency. When code blue is announced, all medical personel immediately spring into action and work together as a team in an attempt to save a life.

Ray Shaw was a conscientious man of high moral character who dearly loved his dog, Shilo. Shilo was a thirty-five pound, slightly overweight Beagle, who had a gentle spirit, and was a pleasure to have as a patient. Shilo was the ideal companion for Mr. Shaw, because her laid back demeanor and complete trust provided him with stress relief. The last thing Mr. Shaw needed in his life was more stress, especially with having a heart condition, and those two were really good for each other.

It was mid-summer when Mr. Shaw called the clinic. He was short of breath, and there was a sense of panic and dread in his voice. "My neighbor just shot my dog in the head, and she's bleeding all over the place. I'm bringing her in right now". Sandy hung up the phone and verbally sounded the alarm, "CODE BLUE! we've got an emergency on the way!" She quickly relayed the nature of the emergency, and all staff members stepped it up a notch, and began preparations for the medical crisis to arrive. Within minutes, Mr. Shaw burst through the clinic door, clutching Shilo in his bloody arms. His face was an ashen-grey color, not good considering his heart condition, and his white T-shirt appeared red because it was saturated with Shilo's blood. She was taken from Mr. Shaw and rushed to the surgery room, while Sandy, a human nurse by profession, assisted Mr. Shaw and his immediate needs. Instead of being faced with one Code Blue, we were confronted with two — Shilo fighting for his life, and Mr. Shaw with his heart condition. It was imperative that cool heads prevailed, and everyone stayed focused!

Shilo's most urgent needs to be addressed were to stop the hemorrhaging and initiate treatment for shock. Once that was achieved and Shilo was stabilized, then the other issues, such as bone fractures and tissue trauma, were assessed. The 22 cal. bullet had entered the left side of Shilo's face, fractured the left mandible (lower jaw bone), and exited the right side of the muzzle, totally obliterating the right mandibular canine tooth and the right mandibular first premolar tooth. There was also extensive soft tissue trauma that would require reconstruction. It was a mess! X-rays revealed that the mandibular fracture was a good candidate for alignment and stabilization with stainless steel wires. The teeth, however, were history. — Gone!

The critical phase of the emergency had passed. Shilo's condition had stabilized, he was no longer in a state of shock, and the hemorrhaging was under control. Mr. Shaw had calmed down, and was less stressed, knowing that his beloved Shilo would survive, but he was still very angry at his neighbor for doing such a heartless thing, —and who could have blamed him.

Due to the compromised bone fractures, Shilo was referred to a veterinary orthopedic surgery specialist, and the surgery went well. The jaw bone fragments were successfully aligned, reunited and stabilized with surgical stainless steel wire, and the soft tissue reconstruction came together nicely. I felt confident that Shilo would make a complete recovery, minus a couple teeth, — and he did.

Looking back, a Code Blue always demands that a team effort be put forth, and our staff handled this one very well, and the outcome was good too. Thanks everybody.

Sweet Success

Veterinary journals and publications provide current and pertinent information pertaining to the diagnosis and treatment of various diseases and maladies. Over the years, I saved and categorized many articles for potential future reference. Several articles were especially intriguing, because they featured the use of honey for the treatment of certain wounds and thermal skin injuries. The results were dramatic and very impressive. It seemed strange, that in today's world of advanced and high-tech medical procedures and treatments, that an age old remedy dating back to the ancient Egyptians, would be revisited. I recalled what Mother used to say, "The proof is in the pudding", and "New is not always better". Those words of wisdom made sense. I was fascinated with the holistic and unconventional treatment method, and hoped that someday I'd have an opportunity to see for myself if treating certain wounds topically with honey really did promote healing.

Perhaps one of the most emotionally gut-wrenching situations for a veterinarian is being confronted with a seriously injured animal, and the owner being financially strapped with extremely limited monetary resources, — i.e. no money. We did have a small compassion fund that was used for hardship cases, but unfortunately, some emergency conditions could have easily depleted that fund. We, as well as all other medical providers, were limited as to how much donated, gratuitous, "free" medical services we could provide. So, — tough, often unpleasant decisions had to be made. Such was the situation encountered with Whitney Mosher and her three year old neutered Pit Bull, named "Tippy".

As I entered the exam room, there was Tippy, laying on the exam table with his weeping owner standing by his side. His left hind leg had been severely traumatized as the result of being bitten by another dog. The skin was badly torn, exposing the underlying muscles and tendons, in two distinct areas between the knee and hip. The four inch long gaping wounds were separated by a mere one inch band of skin. As I was explaining what needed to be done and the surgical reconstruction process, Ms. Mosher tearfully interrupted and said, "Just put him to sleep. I don't have any money, and I can't afford to have anything done for him". I hated the thought of putting Tippy down. There just had to be another way to deal with this problem. Then it hit me, — TRY THE HONEY! I told Ms. Mosher, "I've got an idea. I can't promise anything, and it might be considered "off the wall", by some people, but I think Tippy would be an excellent candidate for the honey treatment. Ms. Mosher looked puzzled until I showed her the veterinary articles and pictures of how honey was used to treat wounds and severe burns on dogs. Her interest instantly peaked when she saw those pictures. I went on to explain that honey was used in ancient times by the Egyptians and the Greeks to treat and heal wounds, and is also being successfully used today in human medicine for certain conditions. Ms. Mosher asked how it worked, and I told her that honey is bactericidal, meaning that bacteria can't live in it, and that's a good thing. I also explained to her that the honey promoted healing by stimulating granulation (the process of filling in with scar tissue). She was now starting to really get excited! I cautioned her that she'd have to be very conscientious about applying the honey twice daily, and that it would be a sticky, messy job,— but it could possibly work if she were willing to put forth the effort. Ms. Mosher smiled and said,

"I'm ok with that! No problem! I'm not working, — so I can be with him all day long if I have to. — I'd be more than willing to do that for my Tippy." Great! Ms. Mosher was given some final instructions, Tippy was placed on oral antibiotics, and now the work began.

Tippy was rechecked weekly for the first three weeks, then every two weeks thereafter. Ms. Mosher was very diligent with Tippy"s honey treatments, and the results were evidence of her commitment. The healing that had taken place after three weeks of treatment was simply astounding! After seven weeks, the wounds were completely healed and barely visible. It was remarkable, — almost unbelievable! Before and after photos, with dates, were taken, and served as proof of the dramatic healing that had taken place, — by simply using HONEY! Tippy was now happy and active again, and Ms. Mosher was elated. The honey treatment was a resounding triumph, and I was looking forward to using it again in the future, — and I did, — and it worked again. Heck, — the honey treatment was, without question, a — SWEET SUCCESS!

Trifecta Plus One

Although the word trifecta is associated primarily with the sport of horse racing, it can also mean three grand events. Cinder may not have been a racehorse, nor were her events all that grand, but they were nonetheless notable because they all occurred within the first year and a half of her life.

Cinder was a very active red siberian husky who loved the freedom and excitement of living in the country. She was, however, a little on the klutzy side, with a persona not unlike that of Inspector Clouseau. Essentially, she was a disaster waiting to happen, and it did.

It all started one summer day when Cinder was in hot pursuit of a rabbit. With reckless disregard for her own safety, she quickly dove under a lowboy trailer in an attempt to catch the prey. Her forehead forcefully struck the metal frame of the trailer, resulting in the tearing back of a large portion of her scalp from her skull. Her owner, Amy Easton, was shocked by what she saw and immediately rushed Cinder to the clinic.

The clinic door swung open and in romped Cinder, with her dislodged scalp waving in the air like a loose toupee tossed in the wind. Cinder didn't display any signs of pain though, in fact, she simply ran directly into the exam room and stood in front of the goodie drawer, waiting for a treat. I grabbed the leash and said to her, "Sorry Cinder, my dear, but we've got to take you to surgery and put you back together, — you know, — and make you pretty again. Okay?" So, down the hall we went, — on our way to a major "make over".

The surgical reconstruction of the failure to duck debacle was, to say the least, very challenging. The point of impact was directly above her eyes. The scalp was peeled backward from that point, going between the ears, and extending to the back of her skull, where it still remained attached. There was only a thin membranous covering left on the skull to serve as an attachment base for the scalp sutures. Reattaching and stabilizing the scalp would prove to be an intricate task. Numerous sutures were delicately placed, — from back to front, — and the end result looked good. Cinder healed very nicely, — all tissue survived, — adhesion was good, and in two weeks post-op, she looked great.

Two months later, Amy called the clinic, and with a voice filled with panic and dread said, "Cinder got her foot caught in a trap or something, and I think she's going to lose her foot. It really looks bad! I'll be in there in a few minutes."

We got all prepared for Cinder, and when she did arrive, she was transported directly into the surgery. Amy was right. It did look bad! The medial (inner) side of her left front paw was severely crushed and mangled, and could not be salvaged. She did lose three digits plus the corresponding metacarpal bones. I was, however, able to save the 4th and 5th digits. She'd still have a paw, albeit half a paw. Cinder was placed on antibiotics and pain medications, and eventually made a successful recovery. I will never cease to be amazed at how rapidly most animals recover and adapt to a major surgical procedure. Cinder acted as if having only half a paw was no big deal. Her indomitable spirit wasn't quenched, and she still retained her zest for life. Cinder was truly an inspiration to all who witnessed her courage, adaptability, determination, and perseverance.

The trifecta was to be completed several months later. Cinder's paw had totally healed, and since she didn't favor the leg at all, it appeared as if nothing had happened. However, Cinder was back to her ole klutzy self.

The old saying, "The road to hell is paved with good intentions", was very apropos in this instance. A hole had been dug to serve as a receptacle for remnants of cut metal, shards of glass, and pieces of conduit and rebar that had accumulated around the ranch. The intent was to safely bury these items and prevent any potential injury to man or beast. The hole, with all it's contents, hadn't yet been covered over with dirt. So, when Cinder went running by, she of course fell in, and was instantly impaled and cut on her right side by the sharp metal and shards of glass. Amy immediately called the clinic, and said that Cinder had, once again, gotten herself in trouble, and needed help. — No kidding!

As usual, Cinder came bounding through the clinic door, and made a beeline for the goodie drawer. She was all happy and playful, seemingly oblivious to her massive wounds. Her right side looked like a jigsaw puzzle of lacerations and punctures, with hair, dirt, debris, and blood mixed within the traumatized tissue. I held her head in my hands and asked her, "Cinder, what in the world did you do this time?" She just looked back at me with those big innocent eyes and continued her incessant tail wagging. That was par for the course with Cinder. So, off to surgery we went — again.

It took three of us, myself and two assistants, over half an hour to irrigate, clean, disinfect, and complete the debridement of nonviable tissue, plus another hour of surgical reconstruction and placement of penrose drains. Our primary concern was embedded contaminants and tissue necrosis (dying and decaying) due to compromised blood supply to certain areas.

When discharging Cinder the next day, I said, "Look Cinder, I really like you, but we've got to stop meeting this way." It sorta went in one ear and out the other. She wouldn't leave the clinic until given another treat. The thought then occurred to me, "Who's being trained here? Me or Cinder?" It appeared to be, —— Moi! The penrose drains were removed the following week, and the surgical site was examined. Miraculously, all the tissue was viable, healing was progressing nicely, and Cinder had once again dodged a bullet. This was now the third major incident for Cinder over the span of a few months, thus completing the trifecta. It's been said that things tend to happen in three's. Well, if that's true, then she shouldn't have much to worry about for awhile.

No more than a month had passed before Cinder was in serious trouble again. Amy called and said, "I think Cinder has really done it this time. She can't stand, can't hold her head up, kinda rolls her eyes like she can't focus, and just lays there. I think she might have broken her neck." When Amy arrived at the clinic, we used a stretcher to transport Cinder from the car to the exam room. Cinder was laying very still, and made a few feeble attempts to raise her head. I tried to get a history from Amy and discussed the possibility of poisonings, and the need for blood analysis, and x-rays. My initial examination revealed no significant abnormalities. Her respirations, mucous membrane color, temperature, pulse, heart rate, and blood analysis results were all essentially within the normal ranges. She didn't exhibit any signs of pain, but she did have delayed muscle reflexes and her eyes were slow tracking. I was just about to take some x-rays of her neck and spinal column, when suddenly she belched. The smell was foul, and strongly resembled the odor of something undergoing fermentation. I asked Amy if Cinder could have possibly eaten some fermenting grain or fruit. She thought for a moment, and then said, "Well, Cinder will eat just about anything, and come to think of it, she's been eating a lot of mule poop lately. My neighbor rides his mules by here just about every day and Cinder goes after that mule poop like it was candy or something. It's gross and disgusting! Could eating that stuff cause a problem?" I told Amy that just about anything was possible with Cinder, but if the mules had been eating a sweet feed that contained grains and molasses, — well, I couldn't totally eliminate that as a possibility. I decided to hospitalize Cinder for observation, and told Amy that I'd give her a report in the morning. As I placed Cinder in the recovery cage for monitoring, she looked up at me, rolled her eyes, and once again made an uncoordinated, feeble attempt to raise her head, then loudly burped. WHEW! It really did smell like something fermented.

As I entered the clinic the next morning, Cinder was right there, standing up, happy as usual, barking for food and attention, and ready to go. No signs of illness or paralysis. Her coordination appeared to be normal, and her eyes were tracking normally as well. Her breath didn't seem to have that fermentation smell either. Could she have tied one on? I couldn't prove it, but all signs were sure pointing in that direction. When Cinder was sent home, I told Amy to keep Cinder away from the mule poop, even if it meant picking it all up, because that poop may have been the culprit. Cinder was kept away from the mule biscuits, and ——— no more problems!

Cinder and her owners moved to Western Washington later that summer, and I lost contact with them. I'd often wondered how klutzy Cinder made it through life. Twenty years had passed, and by some act of providence, I met one of Amy's relatives. I asked the lady about Cinder, and she laughed as she recalled Cinder's accident prone early years. She told me that Cinder lived to be almost 16 years of age, and amazingly, never experienced another accident or serious injury after the move to the coast. That was great, because the Trifecta plus one was enough to last a lifetime.

Lovable, — accident prone, "Cinder"

Murphy

There are many reasons why dogs have been referred to as man's best friend. They are often loyal, devoted, faithful friends and trusted companions who grace us with unconditional love. They become part of us, and when they're no longer here, we can fondly recall those cherished memories that are forever etched in our hearts.

Murphy was an unusual 6 year old Rottweiler. He was a lover, not a fighter, — and he behaved more like a reincarnated lap dog. Instead of having the typical bulky, muscular physique that is usually associated with the Rottweiler breed, Murphy had a long, lean body, with super long legs that actually made him look more like a mini racehorse. He was a good boy who wasted no time zoning in on the "treat" drawer the moment he walked into the clinic. Murphy won me over, and I thoroughly enjoyed having him as a patient.

It was time for Murphy's annual physical exam and vaccinations, and when he walked into the exam room, I noticed him slightly favoring one of his front legs. He looked good physically, — his coat was sleek and shiny, — he had normal heart and lung sounds, and his ears, eyes, nose and throat appeared normal as well. Jeff, Murphy's owner, had been feeding him top quality food, because as Jeff put it, "He's my buddy, and he's worth it!" Jeff was a good and conscientious owner. I asked Jeff if he'd noticed Murphy limping on his left front leg. Jeff said, "Yeah, — he must've sprained it or something." He'd noticed Murphy limping off and on for the last couple of weeks, but didn't think it was that big of a deal. He'd given Murphy an aspirin several times, and that seemed to help. He asked, "Whatcha think it is, Doc?" I told Jeff that there were a myriad of things that could cause a dog to limp. As I began my examination of the leg, I detected a slight swelling on the distal (lower) end of Murphy's radius bone. The swelling was firm, and mildly painful when palpated. I had a bad feeling about that swelling, because osteosarcomas (bone cancer) often appear at that location on the long bones, especially with big dogs. I told Jeff that we needed to take an x-ray of Murphy's leg to see what was going on. Jeff's facial expressions went from cordial to very concerned and serious as he asked, "You don't think it's cancer do you, Doc?" I told him that I couldn't tell for sure without taking an x-ray. I knew, however, that there was a 98% plus chance of it being an osteosarcoma because all the evidence, so far, was pointing in that direction. The x-rays showed an enlargement of the bone on the distal (lower) end of the radius with interruption of the cortex (outer layer) of the bone and secondary bone lysis (disintegration) along with areas of bone deposition. All these findings confirmed my suspicions that Murphy did indeed have bone cancer, and the prognosis was not favorable.

I reviewed the x-rays with Jeff, as Murphy was happily indulging in the treats he was getting from our vet assistant. I explained all of the options available for treatment including chemotherapy, radiation treatments, pain management, amputation, and anti-inflammatory medications. Jeff was numb with shock and disbelief, because sitting next to him was a dog that actually didn't appear sick. He asked, "How much time does Murphy have?" I told him that Murphy had about 6 to 9 months, and even with amputation and chemotherapy, the best scenario wouldn't give him more than one to one and a half years. Jeff definitely needed some time to process the catastrophic situation he was now facing. Several days later, Jeff told me that after a lot of soul searching, he'd come to a decision regarding Murphy. He'd elected to to keep Murphy on pain medications only, allowing his buddy to live free of pain for as long as possible.

Murphy was examined monthly for the next several months. The bone cancer had rapidly grown to the size of a small cantaloupe since first diagnosed six months earlier. Murphy was now unable to use the leg, his appetite had markedly decreased, he'd lost a tremendous amount of weight, and had become very weak. Without question, his quality of life had drastically deteriorated. Murphy had fought the good fight, but the time had come to compassionately relieve him of all the discomfort and suffering.

Jeff requested that Murphy be allowed to cross over at home, and I agreed because transporting Murphy 25 miles would be too stressful for him. Murphy had always liked coming to the vet clinic because he got treats from the "cookie man", —— me. As I entered Murphy's home, I could see him lying there on the sofa, completely stretched out from one end to the other. When he recognized me, his eyes lit up, and with a strong, determined will, he lifted his weak and frail body off the sofa and shuffled across the room on three legs to meet me,— then collapsed. He'd given all he had to come see his ole friend, — "cookie man" Doc. I gave him a cookie/treat that he had come to expect from me, but he only had the strength to take a couple bites. I told him that he'd been such a courageous boy, and that I'd come to help him go to a place where he'd be free from all the pain and where he'd be all healthy again and could run and play all day. I gave him a big hug, and he licked my hand as I told him how much I'd miss him. I then gently and lovingly helped my friend, Murphy, cross over that "Rainbow Bridge".

Perhaps the most difficult task for me to perform as a veterinarian was to put a patient down. I always knew, deep down inside, that I was relieving the pain and suffering, — and that it was, more than anything else, an act of compassion, —but there was always an ache in my heart. God gave us these special friends and faithful four footed companions for a reason — to help us more fully understand the meaning of unconditional love. They have, without a doubt, enriched our lives and will live in our hearts forever.

Mohair Mania

Angora goats are a special breed of domestic goats that were introduced to the United States around 1850. The breed originated in Ankana (Angora) Turkey, and this particular breed of goat is renown for its lustrous, soft hair fiber that's called mohair. They tend to be gentle, delicate animals, and as such, are often vulnerable to predators.

Janice, a former employee, met and married a young dentist, and went on to assist her new husband in his profession. Although not directly involved with veterinary medicine anymore, she still retained her love of animals, all kinds of animals, including her angora goat named "Reddi-Locks".

I'll never forget the day when Janice called the clinic and said that her goat had just been attacked by a dog, and that the little goat's leg was severely injured. When Janice arrived at the clinic, Reddi-Locks was transported straightaway to the surgery room. The little 30 lb. goat was in a state of shock, and that life-threatening condition had to be immediately addressed, before proceeding any further. Dog bite wounds can be very traumatic, but Reddi-Locks' injuries were the worst example of tissue trauma that I'd ever seen! — A mangled mess! The injuries extended from the hoof to a level above her elbow, and went completely around the leg. The skin was shredded, the muscles of the foreleg had been savagely torn to beyond recognition, and there was a high probability of blood vessel and nerve damage. The possibility of saving Reddi-Lock's leg appeared to be extremely remote, and the chance of her ever regaining use of

167

the leg seemed very unlikely. Amputation looked to be the only viable option. Janice understood the gravity of the situation, but nevertheless pleadingly requested that I attempt to salvage the limb, — in spite of the unfavorable odds. I surveyed the mutilated appendage, knowing full well that Janice wouldn't change her mind, so I told her, "Janice, I'll give it my best shot, — it doesn't look very promising, and a lot of things can go wrong, – but maybe we'll get lucky".

Local anesthetics were administered to relieve the pain and discomfort because a general anesthetic would have been too risky, considering Reddi-Locks' compromised condition. Next began the arduous and time consuming task of cleaning all the ground in dirt and embedded hair from the wound. Once that was accomplished, reconstruction was started. The muscles had been ripped, torn across and mangled to such an extent that their identification was nearly impossible. My only recourse was to recall the normal anatomical structures and systematically approximate the muscle pieces according to their size and relative position. Basically, it was an educated guess! Sutures were used to reattach and stabilize the torn sections of muscle, and I did my best to identify and make the proper reconnections. The extent of nerve damage and impairment was difficult to assess. If there were to be any paralysis, it could be either temporary or permanent, depending upon the degree of damage, but only tincture of time would tell. Reconstruction of the macerated skin was the next challenge I faced. Some sections of skin were totally missing, — gone, and some portions had to be removed because they were severely mangled, and their viability was questionable. Many sutures were needed to repair the skin, but eventually that too was completed, and Reddi-Locks looked like she had a leg again, or something that resembled a leg. Lastly, I bandaged the leg, and fabricated a stabilizing splint for her leg and hoof. I modified the bottom of the splint in such a way as to place the hoof in a walking position,

— hoping to restrict movement while the tissue was healing and allow scar tissue to stabilize the carpel joint of the hoof. I cautioned Janice that due to potential nerve and muscle damage, Reddi-Locks would most likely never have tactile sensation to the leg, and she'd probably knuckle over at the carpus for the rest of her life. That would not be good, and if it reached that point, the leg would most definitely have to be amputated. I also told her that I was concerned about having adequate blood circulation to the reconstructed muscles and skin. Poor blood circulation would result in deterioration of the tissue, and that would necessitate removing the leg. —There were a lot of variables, — but we'd just have to wait and see, — cross one bridge at a time.

Reddi-Locks had her bandages changed every few days for the next several weeks, and it was amazing how well the tissue was healing. The pink color of the skin was a good sign, and hair was even beginning to grow. Reddi-Locks was feeling much better overall too, in fact, her appetite was good, and she was even placing weight on the leg. There was also the incessant tapping of her splint on the floor that sounded like a peg-legged pirate was roaming about on the premises.

Four weeks had passed, and it was time to remove the splint. The big questions now were, would there be any paralysis from nerve damage, would she be able to normally place her hoof, or would she need a splint for the rest of her life? When the splint was removed, Reddi-Locks licked her hoof a couple times, and then promptly took off walking down the hallway of the clinic. She was placing her hoof normally, and there was only a slight limp. WOW!

Reddi-Locks steadily improved over the next few months. As her muscles regained their strength, she returned to her usual antics of running all around and jumping up on things. Reddi-Locks had defied the odds. I was totally amazed, — and thankful for her astounding recovery, ————— so was Janice.

"Reddie-locks" enjoying life once again.

Prophetic Words

Fred Macumber was a Pearl Harbor survivor who had devoted his life to the service of his country. This proud man stood 6'4" tall, and towered over his delicately petite wife, Lois, who was barely 5' and probably didn't weigh more than 90 pounds, dripping wet. Fred was always cheerful, spoke with a soft Texas drawl, and doted on his 8 year old Shih Tzu buddy named "Ming".

It was always a pleasure visiting with Fred and Lois when they brought Ming to the clinic for exams and vaccinations. Seeing that tall, slim, happy-go-lucky Texan toting a spoiled little dog in his arms with a quiet, diminutive wife by his side, would make almost anyone smile. It was quite the sight. Fred did all the talking, but Lois controlled the pursestrings, and she knew it too. She was all business, and it didn't take long to figure out who governed that household. Lois may have been small, but inside that little frame was a dynamo.

Ming had been a healthy little guy, so the only time I'd see the Macumbers was when Ming was due for his annual routine check-up. Several years had passed, and the next time Fred brought Ming to the clinic, Lois was conspicuously absent. Fred was more subdued than usual, didn't smile as much as before, and Ming appeared more unkept. I sensed that something wasn't right, and just as I started to examine Ming, Fred said, "You know, I lost my Lois". I told him that I was so very sorry to hear that. Tears welled up in his eyes as he said, "It's really been hard. I miss her so much". He apologized for Ming looking so shabby, but I

171

told him that it wasn't a big deal and that I understood. Losing a spouse can be very devastating, especially after spending so many years together. Fred had lost a soulmate and was overwhelmed with sadness and grief. — It definitely showed. Ming had now become Fred's sole companion, and I was very concerned for both of them.

Six months had passed. It was on a Thursday when Fred called the clinic and told our receptionist that his little dog hadn't been eating for a while, was drinking a lot, vomiting, and now he was just laying around, doing nothing. Ming was put on the daily schedule, and it wasn't long before Fred walked into the clinic, clutching Ming tightly in his arms. I was glad to see that he was accompanied by his eldest son, Mike. Ming appeared listless, depressed, dehydrated, and there was a very strong uremic odor to his breath. Ming's history and symptoms were very suggestive of kidney failure, and the outcome didn't look good for him. I needed to confirm my suspicions, so I drew some blood for analysis. The tests showed elevations of the BUN (blood urea nitrogen), potassium, and phosphorus levels, and he was also anemic. Those results were definite indicators that Ming was in the advanced stages of kidney failure. The prognosis was grave. I explained the results of the tests to Fred and his son, stressed the extreme severity of Ming's condition, and told them that Ming needed to be placed on I.V. (intravenous) fluids and other appropriate medications immediately. Fred then said with fear and desperation in his voice, "Doc, don't let him die, because if he does, — I'll die too". I was stunned by what Fred had just said, because I knew that Ming was in serious trouble, and would very likely die,— regardless of all the treatments. I told Fred and Mike that I'd do my best to save Ming, but he was in the advanced stages of kidney shutdown, and his chances of survival weren't very good.

Ming died the next day, which was a Friday. Four days later, on Tuesday, as I was reading the morning newspaper, I glanced at the obituary column, and —— there it was. Fred Macumber, a Pearl Harbor survivor, had passed away. I was shocked! Fred's prophetic words came flooding over me. He told me he'd die, — and he did! He had lost both of his soul mates, the two who had made his life meaningful, — the two who had given him a reason to live. I truly believe that this gentle man had indeed died of a broken heart.

I asked myself many, many times if there was something more that I could have done, — but there wasn't. I'd come to the realization that I couldn't save them all, no matter how hard I tried. One thing is certain, we should be deeply thankful for our soul mates and companions while they're still with us, — and once they're gone, —we need to hold them gently in our hearts, honor their memory, and love them forever.

Lily

Compassion is defined as concern for the sufferings and misfortunes of others. Not only should compassion be directed towards our fellow man, but also towards our four-footed companions. Strays, abandoned and neglected animals also deserve compassionate care. This humane need prompted us to establish a Compassion Fund that would help provide veterinary care for some of the unfortunate ones.

"Lily"

Lily was a two year old calico farm cat who, according to the owner, hadn't been using her right front leg for three weeks. He wanted her "checked out", but made it perfectly clear that be couldn't afford to spend any money on an ole barn cat. He said that he had a lot of cats around the place, but they'd usually disappear, either wander off or get eaten by the coyotes.

Lily was a beautiful calico cat, and quietly purred as I stroked her head. Her right paw was flexed (curled backward) due to muscle contractions and lack of use of the leg. As I palpated (felt) the leg, movement and swelling could be detected at the midpoint of the humerus bone (upper forelimb bone). I told the owner that the cat's leg was broken, and x-rays needed to be taken to assess the extent of damage. The owner replied, "Forget that! I'll just take her home and she'll have to learn to get around on three legs". I told the guy that she'd be prime coyote bait, but he didn't seem that concerned. I didn't want to see the nice little cat end up that

175

way, so I suggested the possibility of him relinquishing ownership of the cat to me, — I'd then do the surgical repair of the leg and find her a good home where she'd be safe. The man mulled the idea over in his head for a few moments, then quickly signed the transfer of ownership papers, — and left. Lily was now legally mine, — and when all fixed up, she'd at least have a chance to live a "normal" life.

The pre-surgical x-rays revealed a mid-shaft comminuted (many pieces) fracture of the humerus bone, and there were signs indicating that the body was attempting to heal the fractures, but wasn't doing a very good job of it because of instability of the pieces of bone. Lily was taken to surgery where I had to remove many of the unhealthy (nonviable) bone fragments, freshen the ends of the remaining sections of bone, and reunite the bone fragments using stainless steel I.M. (intramedulary) pins and stainless steel circlage wires. It was a lengthy, detailed, often frustrating surgery, but in the end, I was satisfied with the outcome. Lily's leg would be permanently shorter, but she had — "moxie" — she was a boldly determined little girl, and I was confident that she'd do just fine. She recovered from the surgery very nicely, and was a pampered patient throughout her eight week recovery period, and when the the I.M. pin was removed, she started to walk with that leg almost immediately. We'd all become fond of her, and knew that Lily had definitely found a good home, — here, — with us, — as our P.R. clinic cat. It wasn't long before Lily would hop up on the front counter and act as our unofficial greeter. She loved people, and especially loved ladies leather purses. She'd dive right into a handbag and help herself to whatever struck her fancy. It was a riot watching her pull stuff out, — thankfully no one was offended. No doubt about it, she was a real charmer who even licked and groomed some of her most favorite people, — especially Candace. Lily was amazing, — a determined, often headstrong little girl, who learned how to compensate for her shorter front leg, — and actually walked without a limp and jumped like a mini gazelle. Lily really was our little ray of sunshine who brightened our days and was a spoiled member of our staff for many years.

"Lily"

John Deer

When I took the Veterinarian's Oath, I solemnly swore to use my scientific knowledge and skill to relieve animal suffering. The oath, in my opinion, lacked specifics, and was therefore open to interpretation. The State Fish and Wildlife Department had, for whatever reason, authorized only a select few veterinarians to provide veterinary care for wildlife, unfortunately I was not on their list. When presented with a severely injured fawn that the State authorities would have likely to put down rather than treat, I found myself smack dab in an ethical quandary. I asked myself, do I honor my veterinary oath, or do I go along with political correctness protocol? To me, life takes precedence over political correctness, so my decision was easy to make. I was willing to go against the rigid bureaucrats, take a risk, and save a life.

A lady entered the clinic, toting a medium sized dog crate that contained a tiny 20 pound fawn. It appeared amazingly calm, perhaps due to a combination of being overwhelmed with fear and the instinctive behavior of lying perfectly still when injured so as to avoid detection. The fawn had been found entangled in some thick brush near the lady's home. The young deer was most likely running through the brushy forested area and got its' left front leg wedged in the V-shaped section of two diverging branches. When the front knee (carpus) got caught, the momentum of the fawn's body kept going forward, resulting in the knee being almost completely pulled apart. A small band of tendon was the only remaining structure of the knee joint. It was a no-brainer, — the leg had to be amputated.

I anesthetized the fawn, amputated the leg at the level of the knee, and constructed a cushion of soft tissue over the remaining bones. The leg was then bandaged, and the little guy was done. I'd saved a life, and had given the little deer a fighting chance. I felt good about that. The only thing left to do was to give the little guy a name. I started calling him, "John" — you know, — John Deere, — like in tractors.

The next big question was, what do we do with him? Where could we place him so that he could recover safely and secretly? Jill, one of our veterinary assistants, had relatives who lived in a wooded area about eighty miles north. They had a small barn and corral that wasn't being used, and I thought to myself, "That would work perfectly". Now, all we needed to do was to get their permission and cooperation. Contacts were made, and within a couple days, John was on the way to his new home.

As the months passed by, John healed and easily adapted to his new surroundings. He ran, jumped, and played like any other deer, only minus half of a front leg. We were told that he'd occasionally jump out of the corral, go frolic with the other wild deer in the area, then return home and jump back into his corral. John was thoroughly enjoying life again — and his case was a true "feel good" success story.

Today, whenever I see a green John Deere tractor or combine, I don't just see a farm implement, I think of John, the other John Deer, and visualize him running happy and free.

"John" Deer

Mercedes

R andom acts of kindness and concern can restore one's faith in humanity, and in some instances, can even save a life. Such was the case of "Mercedes".

Perhaps the last thing on a person's mind when pulling into a truck stop for gas is to become a hero, of sorts. As fate would have it, while gassing up her car, this business woman saw a young calico cat drop out from the engine compartment of a Mercedes delivery truck that had just pulled up to an adjacent gas pump. The cat appeared dazed and it's face was covered with blood. Forsaking her own time schedule, this good Samaritan took the initiative to seek medical attention for the injured cat. She inquired at the checkout for the location of the nearest veterinarian, who just so happened to be me, and it wasn't long before she burst through the clinic door with the injured cat in hand. As the young cat was being rushed into the exam room, the benevolent stranger made a generous donation to help cover some of the treatment costs, and promptly went on her way, never to be seen again.

The cat was unfortunately another fan belt victim. The entire end of her nose had been torn away, and was barely hanging on by a small strip of skin. She didn't respond to sounds, the pupils of her eyes were dilated, and her body movements were uncoordinated. She had experienced a major blow to the head, and sustained a concussion as well. Instead of referring to her as simply, "cat", we decided to give her an appropriate identity. So, we named her after the make of the delivery truck, "Mercedes".

Mercedes was treated for shock and stabilized before attempting to repair her nose. Veterinary school prepares a person to handle many different medical conditions, but I never thought that I'd be called upon to reattach a nose. These were uncharted waters that I was entering, but I was more than willing to give it a go. I used very tiny 'sutures to reconstruct the nose, and when completed, it looked pretty good. The question now was, would the tissue survive, and would Mercedes' hearing and eyesight improve? Time would tell.

As the days and weeks passed, Mercedes's nose healed remarkably well, and it looked great, — almost as if nothing had ever happened. Her coordination had improved, but her eyesight and hearing problems remained unchanged. My hope was that with tincture of time, there'd be some positive developments. Sandy and the rest of the staff would carry Mercedes with them throughout the clinic as much as possible, but we all realized that Mercedes needed a permanent home. It was decided to place Mercedes on Craig's List as a lovable "special needs" cat. A certain individual involved with a dog rescue program, saw the listing, and told us of her friend who operated a "special needs" cat rescue in the city of Ellensberg, about 170 miles away. It was essentially a cat ranch for disabled felines. That was the perfect place for Mercedes! We contacted them, discussed Mercedes' case, and they agreed to accept her into their facility. They already had several deaf and blind cats at the "ranch", so they were familiar with handling cats with those types of disabilities. Arrangements were made, and Mercedes was transported to her new home.

The owner of the special needs cat ranch was wonderful. She sent us periodic pictures of Mercedes, and updates on her condition. As time passed, her hearing and eyesight did improve, and she was once again enjoying life. She fit in nicely, got along well with all the other cats, and eventually Mercedes became the queen of the household. We couldn't have been happier for Mercedes. It is definitely true, — random acts of kindness can indeed bring joy.

Sweet little "Mercedes"

Sammy

Animals can teach us many things about life in general, — but we must be observant and perceptive. Adaptability, resilience, and perseverance are several attributes that come to mind when I recall a little cat named Samantha ("Sammy"). Her indomitable spirit enabled her to rise above her disability to live a relatively normal, happy life.

Sammy was presented to the veterinary clinic with a horrendous ear mite infestation involving both ears. Ear mites can be very irritating to the patient, because the little guys burrow down into the ear canal tissue and produce intense itching. The patients will respond by doing the obvious, — they instinctively scratch and rub at their ears almost non-stop. This response further complicates the situation by introducing bacteria to the already irritated and inflamed tissue. In some advanced cases, the ear mites and infection can penetrate deeply into the middle and inner ear. Not a good situation, because the inner ear houses the cochlea and semicircular canals which act somewhat like a gyroscope to help regulate equilibrium and influence balance. When or if they're damaged, the effects are often irreversible. Unfortunately, such was the case with Sammy.

The owner had been battling the ear mite problem for quite a while, periodically using OTC (over the counter) ear mite preparations from discount stores. She hadn't seen much, if any improvement. Her main concern at this point was the tremor-like head bobbing and equilibrium issues that the cat was experiencing. I explained the complexity of the situation, and the distinct possibility that the inner ear could be permanently affected. That didn't go over very well with the owner! She emphatically told me that she'd had enough, wasn't going to spend any more money on the cat, and just wanted me to put the cat down. I told her that I wouldn't do that, but, if the ownership of the cat was signed over to me, I would treat the cat and find it a good home. The lady signed the transfer of ownership papers without hesitation, and was gone. I looked down at the sweet little bobble-headed cat, and said to her, "Sammy, you're mine now, so let's see what I can do for you,— okay.?"

The next day Sammy was placed under general anesthesia so that her ears could be painlessly cleaned and treated. Her ear mite infestation and ear infection resolved, but as expected, her equilibrium issues persisted. Sammy was destined to have balance challenges for the rest of her life, but I knew she'd make it, because she impressed me as being a survivor, a real overcomer. The amazing thing about Sammy was that her disability bothered other animals more that it bothered her. She was essentially a normal cat who unfortunately possessed some major locomotion issues. When she would get excited or tried to chase and play with other animals, her head wobbling and leg flailing really intensified. Sometimes she'd actually lose her balance and fall over on her side, but she handled it like a pro. She'd collect herself, and get right back up. Heck, she acted like it wasn't such a big deal, only a minor inconvenience. That resilient little charmer had a lot of hutzpah.

Sammy liked everybody, and she assumed that everybody liked her too, and wanted to play. So, it wasn't unusual to see her take off in her "wild" and unorthodox gallop towards some unsuspecting dog or cat. Her head would shake like some bobble-head doll, and her legs would gyrate in all directions. She may have thought that she was in control, but nobody else did. Most of the animals just froze, startled and bewildered at the sight of this whirling dervish coming kind of straight at them. Many couldn't process the weird sight, and took off running in the opposite direction, but a few seemed amused by her unorthodox movements, — let her approach, and some even played with her. You know, — different strokes for different folks!

It wasn't long before a client told his son and daughter-in-law about the sweet "special needs" cat at the vet clinic that needed to find a loving home. The young couple stopped by to see Sammy and were instantly smitten with her. It was a perfect match in many ways. Sammy had found the home that she really needed, — and deserved.

Sammy is a real success story of a cat with a disability, who when given a chance, showed how she could adapt to and overcome her handicap. She continues to improve and now can even jump up on furniture and scold the birds outside the window. Sammy has brought love and joy to her new home, and she continues to be an inspiration to all who are fortunate enough to meet her.

"Sammy", a true inspiration

Alternatives

The ancient healing art of acupressure and its use in veterinary medicine had been a subject of interest to me for many years. When the opportunity presented itself, I enrolled in an acupressure class in Colorado to receive formal training. After completing the course, it didn't take long before I was presented with a case where I could apply my newly acquired skills.

A lady entered the clinic with a young black kitten cradled in her arms. She'd found the kitten laying in the middle of a secondary county road, unable to use it's left hind leg. It was her compassion for animals that prompted her to rescue the little guy and get him to a veterinarian for medical treatment. She told Megan, our receptionist, that she was on her way to work, and wasn't able to keep the cat, but was willing to make a donation to our Compassion Fund. She then thanked us, and went on her way.

Sitting there nonchalantly on the exam table was a young, 4 month old, black kitten with big gold eyes, seemingly UNDERwhelmed by all that was taking place around him, and showing absolutely no signs of pain or discomfort. The initial exam showed no evidence of any wounds, scrapes, bruises, or broken bones. The left hind leg, unfortunately, appeared to be paralyzed. The leg muscles were flaccid (limp) and unresponsive to the toe pinch-reflex test. The leg was non-weight bearing, the righting-reflex of the paw was absent, but the blood circulation to the leg appeared to be normal. X-rays confirmed that there were no vertebral or pelvic abnormalities. All the findings were pointing towards a major nerve injury, specifically the sciatic nerve and its branches. Such nerve injuries usually do not improve, and the affected limb remains permanently paralyzed and non-functional. The conventional treatment protocol for such injuries was amputation. I paused for a moment, and was considering my limited treatment options, when Sandy, our office manager, interjected with a pivotal question, "Would that acupressure point therapy help in a case like this?". I said, "Good question. Let's take a look.". I quickly checked my references for any acupressure points that could benefit hind leg paralysis cases. VIOLA! There they were! I made diagrams of the specific point locations, and proceeded to teach the vet assistants how to stimulate the designated points. I explained that this alternative therapy regime was definitely a long shot, and I needed to have everyone actively involved. Everybody came on board, and we were now, good to go.

The kitten, who we named "Panther", was scheduled for acupressure point stimulation twice daily. Pinch-reflex test responses and righting-reflex responses were to be monitored and recorded daily as well. In addition, I placed Panther on a holistic oral supplement that stimulated the release of his own stem cells into his circulatory system to aid tissue repair. Panther thoroughly enjoyed his treatment sessions, and all the attention. He thought the sessions were just a special time to play "scratch and tickle". Two weeks of dedicated treatments had been completed without seeing any response whatsoever. Even though our efforts hadn't produced any positive results, we still remained committed to completing an entire month of treatments before reassessing the case. When the pinch-reflex test was performed during the third week of treatment, Panther's toes moved ever so slightly and his paw retracted a tiny bit. The spontaneous hoots and hollers of joy that erupted from the staff actually startled poor little Panther. He wasn't frightened for long because he was quickly smothered with petting and praises of, "Good Boy, Panther". Over the next two weeks, his responses to the pinch-reflex test continued to improve and get stronger, — and by the seventh week, Panther was able to successfully place his paw and support weight. A week later he was walking on the leg, and the following week, Panther astonished us all by running down the hallway, albeit with a limp. From that point on, it was, "Katie bar the door". Panther's new found confidence transformed him from a laid-back little guy into a thrill seeker who had to be up and on anything and everything. That was the not-so-subtle clue that Panther needed to find a permanent home. Since many people had been watching Panther's progress and were enamored with his "Little Engine That Could" personality, it was an easy task to place him. In fact, within days he'd found a loving home just six blocks from the clinic.

Panther was my first acupressure therapy patient, and I was very pleased with the outcome. I'd found that alternative therapies can afford viable options of treatment in veterinary medicine, and Panther was a prime example.

"Panther"

Little Willow

The road of life can have many ups, downs, twists and turns. Getting lost or sidetracked along the way can pose some very difficult challenges. Such was the case with a small Scottish Fold cat.

It was impossible to know where the cat's journey began. What is known is that the original owner named the cat, "Heath", but couldn't care for it. She gave the cat to a young lady named Crystal, who lived in a small apartment, and was financially strapped herself. Being unemployed, Crystal had to move back home to live with her parents. During the move, the cat somehow got away and disappeared. Crystal went back to the apartment several times, and looked for Heath, but couldn't find him. Three weeks later a neighbor found the cat huddled in a stairwell. He had lost a lot of weight, was very frightened, and refused to eat. Crystal knew something was wrong and that Heath needed some medical help right away, so she called the clinic.

Crystal placed the thin, anorexic, and scared grey tabby cat on the examination table. The 2 year old cat was rather small, only about five pounds. As I raised its tail to insert the thermometer, I noticed that the plumbing was that of a female, not a male. I said to Crystal, "Did you know that you have a female here". Crystal replied, "Really! We didn't ever see him come into heat, so we thought that he was a male. No wonder". She laughed sheepishly, then said, "Wow, that's weird". I told Crystal that we needed to give "her" a more feminine name, so we came up with, "Willow".

Willow possessed the typical folded-over ears that are characteristic of the Scottish Fold breed. Her legs were shorter than most
cats, and her joints were visibly swollen, deformed, and not very
flexible when manipulated. Willow, unfortunately, had osteochon-
drodysplasia, a hereditary disease that is unique to Scottish Folds.
The condition can produce a severe crippling lameness early in
life, and in time, progresses to a full blown, painfully debilitating
arthritis. Willow's life was destined to be an agonizing struggle.

Willow had many issues going on. I told Crystal that first of all,
blood tests would be needed to assess the health state of Willow's
internal organs, and testing for feline leukemia and feline im-
munodeficiency disease were also very important. Willow was
severely dehydrated and would need to be placed on I.V. fluids,
plus she'd need nutritional supplementation and pain medications
for her arthritic joints. X-rays were also recommended to evaluate the heart, lungs, and internal organs for any abnormalities
and tumors indicative of cancer. Poor Crystal was overwhelmed
by what she'd heard. She told me that she liked the cat, but was
financially unable to do anything for Willow. Then Crystal asked,
"What should I do? — Should I put her out of her misery? I don't
want to see her suffer this way." I told Crystal that Willow was an
exceptional little girl with a sweet spirit, but regrettably she possessed a fragile little body. "Crystal", I said, "What do you think
about the clinic becoming Willow's new permanent home? We
would do all the testing and treatments, and if the test results were
negative and if she responded to the treatments, then she could
stay here. She'd live in a safe place, get lots of attention, get her
daily treatments, and have all her needs met." You could almost
see the heavy burden of concern lift from Crystal's shoulders.
Crystal smiled and said, "Yes. That would be good. Let's do that."

Willow was a good patient. She successfully made it through
the initial testing and therapy, and then became one of our clinic

cats. She had her own quiet place, a soft therapeutic bed, specially formulated food for arthritic conditions, and she also received an array of medications, injections, and nutraceutical supplements to ease her arthritic pain. Willow responded really well! She gained weight, and there were times when she even felt good enough to play. She was finally enjoying life, and everyone loved her.

Two years had passed, and Willow had been living a sheltered life. Then she began to slowly loose weight, her appetite decreased, and she become less active. Her trips to the water bowl had also increased. Those patterns of behavior raised a red flag, and prompted us to run some blood tests and take x-rays of her abdomen. Her BUN (blood urea nitrogen) and creatinine levels were abnormally high, and the x-rays showed that her kidneys were enlarged. Not a good sign. An ultrasound was scheduled and performed, and it showed that her kidneys had many fluid filled cysts, — polycystic kidney disease was confirmed. It was a problem frequently encountered with the Scottish Fold breed. How can kidneys function this way? The answer, — they can't! The handwriting was on the wall, and it was just a matter of time.

All efforts were used to make Willow as comfortable as possible throughout her final days, but the eventual outcome was inevitable. We had given little Willow as good a life as could have been expected, considering the circumstances. The courage and gentleness that she showed throughout her short life would forever be a source of inspiration to all who knew and loved her.

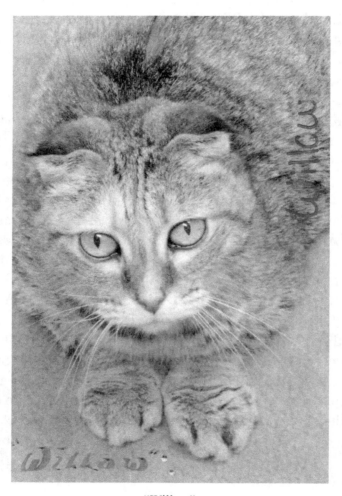

"Willow"

Bartering

B artering is an age-old process involving the exchange of goods and services without the use of money. It is an arbitrary transaction, and the items bartered can range from the ridiculous to the sublime. It has been said, and inferred, that beauty as well as value, is in the eye of the beholder, and I'd found that to be very true. Our intent was to essentially hold the bartered item as collateral until the incurred veterinary bill was paid in full. Most of the items were returned to the owners, but there were occasions where the bartered items were never reclaimed. The scenario that usually existed involved an animal that needed veterinary care and an owner with very limited or no finances.

Over the years, we held radios of all makes and sizes, and occasionally a nice boom box was bartered. Most of the items were of excellent quality and worked well. We also received an assortment of power tools, wrenches, and socket sets, — very useful things, but as expected, they were always reclaimed. One of the most unusual items bartered was an old saddle. It didn't look like much, but it was a prized possession to the owner. I thought that I'd be stuck with an old, dirty, smelly saddle, but the guy paid off his veterinary bill within two months, and took off with his treasure, — thank goodness.

It was always interesting to see what people offered as collateral to cover their bills. There were rings, wrist watches, and even car titles. One particular client, who just so happened to be an artist, asked me if I'd be willing to trade veterinary services for an oil painting of Mikey, our clinic cat. I told her, "Sure"! I'd known Mrs. Collins for many years, had seen her work, and it was very good. Several weeks had passed and then one day Mrs. Collins came walking into the clinic with a 14x16 inch framed oil painting of Mikey in hand. Her face beamed with pride as I hung the painting on the hallway wall. She stepped back, cocked her head to one side, and suddenly her smile turned into a frown as she said, "There's something wrong with that painting. It just doesn't look right." I took a closer look, and said to Mrs Collins, "Mikey doesn't have a nose". "You're right!" She said. "I forgot to finish his nose. Heck, we can't have that. I'll just have to take him back home with me and give him a proper nose. How did I ever miss that?" Well, it wasn't long before she returned with the finished product. Mikey now had a nose, the painting looked complete, and adorned the clinic hallway wall for many years to come.

We've all heard the old saying, "You can't judge a book by it's cover". That adage perfectly applied to Ms. Tremble. Ms. Tremble had two cats that needed to be checked over, wormed, vaccinated, and treated for fleas. She was a very imposing woman, tall, broad shouldered, ruddy weathered complexion, and wore a man's red plaid long sleeved shirt outside of her jeans. As she placed the cats on the exam table, she asked, "Would you be willing to trade services? — I don't have much money". If there was ever such a thing as a female Paul Bunyan, she was it! I didn't want to tick off this person, so I said, "Uh, sure. What do you have?". "Canned goods and preserves", she replied. I told her that would be great, but honestly, I had some major reservations. She asked me how much I needed, and I told her that she could bring in as much as she thought was fair. She nodded approval and said that she'd bring the goods by the next day. I then continued to work on her cats and asked myself, "What have you gotten yourself into now?"

The following day Ms. Tremble entered the clinic toting two huge cardboard boxes. She placed them on the exam table and said, "I hope this is enough". As she gently removed the contents of the boxes and placed them on the table, my eyes almost popped out of my head. There before me were jars and jars of the most beautiful and perfectly prepared fruits, vegetables, and preserves that I'd ever seen. Each container could have easily won top honors at any state fair in the country! The colors, the clarity, the arrangement of the contents was absolutely flawless! I was astounded! I complemented Ms. Tremble on her work, and told her that these weren't just canned goods, they were works of art. She smiled and her rosy cheeks blushed a little. She was proud of her work, and pleased that someone appreciated all her devoted and painstaking efforts. I'd learned a valuable lesson that day, — never prejudge people and their abilities.

The bartering process had proven to be fun, interesting, and profitable. It turned out to be a win-win situation for everyone involved, but most importantly, the animals received the medical care they needed.

Cedar

The rising morning sun heralded the beginning of a new day of challenges and opportunities. A person had to be mentally and emotionally prepared for what lay ahead, because the ensuing day could to be a roller coaster of events filled with triumphs and and tragedies, — but such is the life of a veterinarian.

Allergic reactions to certain foods and plants had been a lifelong battle for me. I'd experienced periodic episodes of severe skin irritation, inflammation, rashes and itching. Dietary restrictions, oral medications and nutritional supplements helped to moderate the problem, but acupuncture therapy was very helpful in providing relief. I'd made an appointment for an acupuncture treatment, and while sitting in the waiting room, I heard the muffled lonesome whines of a dog in the adjacent room. I got up from the chair and went to investigate what kind of dog was making those forlorn sounds. As I peered over the door gate, there he sat, a big, handsome, well groomed Golden Retriever. I looked down at him and said, "Hey buddy, what's your name?" At that very moment, the acupuncturist, Ms. Jessup, opened the door to the waiting room, and walked over to the dog and said, "Cedar, you know better than that. Stop your whining." I asked, "Is he your dog?" Ms. Jessup responded, "Yes, —— he is — and he knows that he's supposed to be quiet. He's a very good boy most of the time, but once in a while he gets a little lonesome. Cedar was now standing up, wagging his tail, and had that happy-go-lucky smile look on his face. You could tell by the looks exchanged between Ms.

Jessup and Cedar that there was a very strong bond between those two. I usually carried dog treats in my car, so I asked Ms. Jessup if I could give Cedar few treats. She gave the okay. I ran to the car, grabbed a couple treats, and rushed back to a patiently waiting, enthusiastic Cedar. He chowed down the goodies, and now we were bosom buddies for life. He quickly became my shadow, accompanied me to the therapy room and patiently sat by my side throughout the acupuncture session. That scenario was to be repeated many times over the next several months of treatments, and during that time, Cedar and I forged a strong friendship.

It was a warm Wednesday afternoon in June that I'd scheduled an appointment with Ms. Jessup for another acupuncture treatment. Cedar of course, had to get his treat and be there with me during my session. Ms. Jessup had just finished inserting the acupuncture needles all over my body, and then she told me that Cedar needed to go for a short walk, and that they'd only be gone a few minutes. She asked me if I'd mind being by myself . Heck, I didn't mind, — so off they went. I was just laying there, listening to the soothing music, — when suddenly I heard the sharp screeching of tires — then a dull thud. I will never forget that sound! It wasn't the characteristic metallic sound one would expect from two cars colliding, — it was more muffled. My immediate thoughts were that perhaps a pedestrian or someone on a bike got hit, or maybe a dog. — Then I remembered that Cedar had gone on a walk, — I hoped that it wasn't him, — but I had that sick feeling in the pit of my stomach. Suddenly Ms. Jessup came bolting into the treatment room. Her face was pale and she was visibly shaking. She started frantically pulling the acupuncture needles from my body, and with a trembling voice she said, "Cedar just got hit by a car. He slipped out of his collar and ran out into the street — it happened so fast! —I gotta go!" Then off she ran. I immediately jumped off the table, tossed on my white

T-shirt, and jetted out of the building in my running shorts and barefoot. There in the middle of a very busy 4-lane street lay Cedar. The traffic had come to a standstill, and many of the on-lookers appeared stunned and deeply concerned. I ran to Cedar, oblivious to the cars and moving traffic, got down on my knees next to Cedars's motionless body, and immediately started giving him CPR, and even attempted mouth to mouth resuscitation. He didn't look good, — he was slipping away. I kept telling him to stay with me, but all my efforts were in vain. He wasn't breathing on his own, and I watched the pupils of his eyes slowly dilate and become fixed. As the pink color of his gums slowly turned ashen-pale, — I knew he was gone. —— It happened so fast! — I tried, — did the best I could, but wasn't able to save my buddy. I closed his eyes, stroked his head, and told him that I was so very sorry that I couldn't help him. I then lifted his lifeless body into my arms and carried him from that surreal scene. My T-shirt, hands and face were covered with Cedar's blood, and I felt a numbing sense of loss. It all seemed like a cruel nightmare and I just wanted to wake up and it would all be gone, — but it wasn't. The day had started out so good, but ended up being truly heart wrenching.

Throughout the years, whenever I'd see a Golden Retriever, I'd be reminded of my very special friend, Cedar. We sure enjoyed each others company, and one thing was certain, — I was there with him at the end, and I even carried him home.

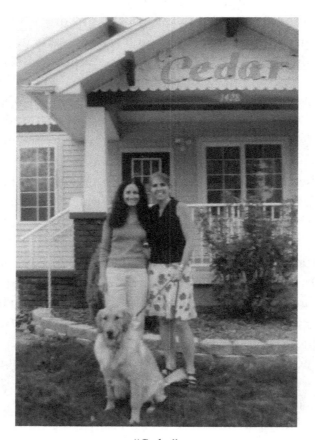

"Cedar"

Reggie

The anatomy classes in veterinary school demanded many hours of intense study and memorization. All that hard work and effort paid off, especially when confronted with cases involving severe traumatic wounds that left structures so terribly damaged that they were almost unrecognizable.

The man on the phone simply said that his dog had been shot in the leg, and he thought it needed to be checked out. When the Rottweiler-cross canine walked into the clinic, he was holding up his right hind leg. His owner appeared to be disgusted and inconvenienced with the whole situation, and really didn't seem all that concerned. He actually thought that the wound would heal on its own, but his girlfriend convinced him to at least have it checked out. There was a large amount of dried blood on the leg, causing heavy matting of the medium length hair, and obscuring the true extent of the injury. The owner was told that his dog, named "Reggie", had to be placed under a general anesthesia so that the wound could be thoroughly cleaned, debrided, and treated without inflicting any more pain. The owner grudgingly consented.

Once the hair was shaved and the matts removed, it was plain to see that Reggie had been shot most likely with a smaller caliber hollow point bullet. There was a small point of entry hole on the back of his leg, midway between his knee and hip. It was obvious that Reggie had been somewhere where he shouldn't have been, and was shot as he was running away. X-rays revealed no broken bones, the bulk of the bullet had exited, but there were remnants of the projectile dispersed throughout the muscle tissue. The bullet had miraculously missed the major arteries, veins, nerves, and the femur bone as well, but there was massive muscle damage as the bullet exited out the front of his thigh. Hollow point bullets tend to mushroom out, tumble and deviate upon entry. Such projectiles grab and rip tissue, — and produce huge exit wounds. Reggie had large hunks of disfigured quadriceps muscle protruding from the six inch wide hole in his leg. The quadriceps muscle is made up of four subdivision muscles, which control the extension of the knee (stifle). The torn, mangled, and severed muscles had to be identified and reattached to their corresponding members in order for Reggie to have any hope of walking or even running normally again. It was a long and tedious surgery, but when finished, I was confident that all the muscles had been correctly reunited. Reggie now had a very good chance of making a complete recovery, and he did just that.

It had all worked out well for Reggie. There was, however, one major fly in the ointment, — we did not get paid for our services, — not a red cent, — NOTHING, — ZIPPO! The owner walked out on his bill, — flooped the coop, — bailed out, — left the area. I would never see Reggie again, — but I knew, deep down inside, that I'd done my best to help that dog, — and my efforts had allowed him to once again walk and run free. — I could live with that!

A Movie Made the Difference

I can't remember the name of the movie, but there was one particularly graphic scene that stuck in my mind. The movie was set in medieval England, around the 1400's, during the reign of King Arthur. There was a pregnant young maiden who'd been in labor for a very long period of time, and due to complications of childbirth, was nearing death. An old peasant midwife was summoned, but she arrived at the castle a moment too late. The young maiden had just drawn her last breath, and died. The old woman entered the room, saw the dead maiden, and immediately yelled, "We must save the child!". Then, without a moment's hesitation, she grabbed a large knife and proceeded to perform the fastest and most crude caesarian section that I'd ever seen. She'd rescued a live infant from a lifeless mother. That was a shocking and very troubling scene to view, and one which I'd never forget.

The owners of a very pregnant Dachshund named "Tilly" had left on vacation, and asked their neighbor, Karen, to care for and supervise Tilly in their absence. Karen called the clinic that fateful day, and with a voice filled with concern and trepidation said, "I'm caring for my neighbor's pregnant dog, and she started pushing to have puppies a couple days ago, and now nothing is happening, — she's just laying there, barely breathing, and I think she's dying." Kathleen, our receptionist, told Karen to get Tilly to the clinic as fast as possible, because the dog was in serious trouble. Karen arrived within a few minutes, entered the clinic carrying a lifeless, pregnant dachshund, and was speedily ushered to the surgery room. Tilly's pupils were fully dilated and fixed, there was no heartbeat, but her body was still warm. She had just died! At that very moment, I recalled the morbid movie scene from years past. I quickly grabbed a scalpel, made a swift incision down her swollen abdomen, exposed and elevated the enlarged uterus, made another incision, and proceeded to remove three seemingly lifeless puppies. I quickly handed the lifeless puppies, one by one, to the vet assistants, and within seconds the puppies were being resuscitated. Believe me, there is no sweeter sound than the first cries of a newborn. Soon Sandy chimed out, "This one's starting to breathe!", and then it cried. That really got everyone excited! It didn't take long before the puppy Vicky was working on started breathing too. The third puppy, however, didn't respond.

The two surviving puppies had to be hand raised, but eventually they grew up to be very healthy, spoiled, little wiener dogs. It was truly rewarding to see them escape the grip of death and grow up to enjoy life. I'd often think about those puppies, how their lives were in such extreme peril, and that they were literally within seconds of dying. I needed to make a quick decision at a very critical moment, and oddly enough, the disturbing movie scene that was etched in my mind,—— made the difference! Basically, each of us is the summation of our experiences, and those experiences can, and do, influence our behavior and actions, — actions that someday might make the difference between life and death.

A Wild Experience

The time had come for the vinyl flooring in the waiting room to be replaced. We'd looked at many samples, and finally selected a nice commercial grade linoleum that promised to meet our needs. We didn't, however, anticipate that the new flooring would be so thoroughly tested the day after installation.

Mrs. Schaeffer had arrived a few minutes early for her 9:00 A.M. appointment, and was patiently sitting in the waiting room with her recently groomed little Pomeranian, "Lady". Mrs. Schaeffer was an older German woman who was always punctual, and fastidious about her home, her appearance, and her dog. The clinic door suddenly swung open wildly, and a 130 pound Nubian goat standing about 30 inches at the withers, came charging into the waiting room with its owner, Betty Jones, in tow on the lead rope. She hadn't made an appointment, and assumed that she could just walk in the front door with her goat. Mrs. Jones blurted out, "Can you take a look at my goat's bag? I think she has mastitis or something else going on down there. It feels warm". Just as Donna, our receptionist, was telling Mrs. Jones that we couldn't examine a farm animal in the waiting room, but we could out back, the goat CUT LOOSE! It raised its tail, semi-squatted, and peed a lake! Urine flew all over the place, and then the goat pooped! After TOTALLY relieving itself, the goat started swinging around the waiting room on its lead, stepping in and kicking poop pellets soaked in urine everywhere. Poor Mrs. Schaeffer, she sat there with goat pee and poop all over her ankles and shoes, a disgusted expression on her face, and a protective grip on little Lady. As Betty Jones and her goat were being ushered out the door, and to the back of the clinic, Betty casually said, "I'll help clean up this place." I examined the goat out back of the clinic while some of the staff members attended to cleaning up the waiting room, — and Mrs. Schaeffer. As I was finishing up with the goat, Mrs. Jones nonchalantly said, "Oh, — I left home so fast that I forgot my purse. — Just send me a bill." She then loaded the goat into her pickup, and took off. She'd left us with a waiting room full of goat feces and urine, and a client who was almost in a state of shock after enduring the horrendous "voiding goat" experience.

Our new floor had been baptized, not by fire but by goat poop and pee. Thankfully the weather was warm, because all doors and windows had to remain open for the remainder of the day, just to air-out the clinic. We did manage to eventually get the waiting room clean, and the new flooring had withstood the test with flying colors.

Never a Dull Moment

Some jobs and professions can be dull, boring, and unfulfilling, but not veterinary medicine. If variety is supposed to be the spice of life, then veterinary medicine is a well seasoned profession. Unusual cases, unexpected events and situations made life very interesting and challenging. There was never a dull moment, because no two days were ever the same, — and that was the "New Normal".

The Tail

The color of paint chosen for the clinic waiting room was called Navajo White. It was a pleasant off-white neutral color that went well with the wooden paneling and burnt orange colored chairs. Sandy and I did the painting after hours on the weekend, and there was still a faint new-paint smell when we opened the clinic for business the following Monday.

A young lady called and scheduled an appointment to have her Russian Borzoi's tail "checked". She said that the end of the dog's tail had gotten slammed in the door, and she'd managed to apply a bandage to stop the bleeding. Now, Russian Borzois are large dogs that possess long, skinny tails and it was understandable how something like this could happen. As the lady entered the clinic, she proceeded to praise the dog for being such a good boy, and he responded by wildly wagging his long thin tail. The centrifugal force generated from the vigorous tail wagging caused the bandage to immediately fly off, exposing the bloody tail, which instantly started to actively bleed again. The dog was, by nature, a happy, excitable guy, and the more the owner consoled him, the more he wagged his tail, and the more it bled. Blood was soon being flung everywhere throughout the room, —— on the floor, up the walls, and even across the ceiling. Our newly painted waiting room now looked like a macabre work of modern art.

The dog was quickly restrained, and the tail was examined. The tip of the tail had been severely crushed and there was major tissue damage. The only viable option of treatment in this case was amputation of the end of the tail. The surgical procedure took approximately thirty minutes to complete, but it took three people more than two hours to clean the blood spattered waiting room. Thank heavens we used a paint that was capable of being washed.

The Lucky Pup

Angela, our receptionist, hung up the phone and promptly announced, "There's a guy coming in with his puppy that's just been attacked by an eagle." I'd never heard of anything like that happening in this area before, so maybe the owner was mistaken. Anyway, we'd find out shortly.

It wasn't long before the owner arrived at the clinic, and was ushered into the exam room with a frightened twelve week old, sixteen pound Black Labrador puppy cradled in his arms. I asked the owner if he was sure that it was an eagle that attacked his pup, and the owner responded, "Heck yes I'm sure! —— I saw it happen! The eagle tried to grab both pups, but as he tried to take off with a pup in each claw, the weight must have been too much for him, so he dropped this pup, and flew off with the other one". As I examined the puppy, the talon marks were glaringly obvious on the puppy's sides. There was no doubt! Only a huge bird, like an eagle, could make puncture wounds like that.

The puppy was anesthetized, and his wounds were cleaned, treated, and sutured. Thankfully the talons had not penetrated the thoracic or abdominal cavities. The little guy was fortunate to be alive. He healed nicely, made a total recovery, and always kept a weary eye looking upward, ever vigilant for any danger that might be looming overhead.

A Real Survivor

A strong "will to live" is a powerful force that can literally determine whether an individual lives or dies. This phenomenon can be seen with animals as well as people, and witnessing its impact can be an amazing and often inspiring experience.

A little white eight month old miniature poodle named "Alice" had been sick for two days. According to the owners, Alice was vomiting, had bloody diarrhea, wasn't eating, and appeared weak. When the owner arrived at the clinic, they carried a prone, motionless Alice on a plywood board into the first exam room. At first glance, she appeared totally lifeless, but then she made a feeble gasp. Alice was extremely weak, there was blood-tinged vomit stuck to the hair around her mouth, she was severely dehydrated, and watery foul smelling bloody diarrhea was oozing from her rectum. She was in tough shape, and this definitely looked like a Parvo case. She appeared to be on her way out, and in instances like this, euthanasia would have been considered an act of kindness. I was just about to recommend that option to the owners, but first I leaned over, patted her on the head and told her, "Alice, you gotta help me get you through this. — Okay?" As weak and sick as this dog was, she struggled to raise her little head and looked me straight in the eyes. That's all I needed to see! She may have been very close to death, but there was that undeniable "will to live" glint in her eyes. I told the staff, "Let's go for it, —— this little lady has a chance, —— she wants to live!"

Everyone jumped into action. It was a real team effort. Blood was drawn for tests, I.V.'s were placed, and life-saving fluids flowed into her veins. Antibiotics and gastrointestinal sedatives and protectants were also given while other staff members cleaned up Alice's soiled little body. The tests confirmed that Alice did indeed have Parvo, a severe hemorrhagic enteritis condition where the Parvo virus attacks and destroys the mucosal lining of the intestinal tract. It is a very serious disease which often results in death.

Alice's response to the treatment was utterly amazing! Within hours she was sitting up and wagging her little stump of a tail. She continued to receive I.V. fluid therapy for the next 24 hours, and the following day was discharged with specific medications and instructions. Alice's complete recovery was a testament to her strong will to live, and she proved that little miniature poodles can be pretty tough customers. Alice was, without a doubt, "A Real Survivor".

A Common Bond

A good samaritan brought two recently orphaned white short-hair kittens to the clinic, hoping that we could find them good homes. The mother cat had been hit by a car and died, leaving the kittens to fend for themselves. Since that time, they had sought refuge under the lady's deck. These two bright eyed, frightened little orphans needed some help, and I reassured the lady that we'd take the kittens and do our best to place them in loving homes. She smiled, thanked us, and went on her way.

The first order of business was to give these eight week old kittens a thorough physical exam, then deworm and vaccinate them. These little tykes appeared well fed, thanks to the concerned lady, and they were also free of ear mites and fleas. So far, so good. Their eyes were clear, their temperatures were within normal limits, and they had normal lung sounds, but — the tiny female had a very distinct heart murmur. It was congenital, and most likely a mitral valve or septal defect. There was an outside chance of some improvement with tincture of time, but that possibility was highly unlikely. The bottom line was that this little girl would need special care, including heart healthy diets, heart medications, and supervised activity. She could, however, live an essentially normal life, but in all likelihood, her lifespan would be shortened. It would certainly be a challenge to find a suitable home for a kitten who was clearly behind the 8-ball.

It didn't take long for the staff to come up with names for the duo. The little boy was named, "Marshmellow", and the tiny girl was given the fitting name, "Cotton". We monitored the kittens health for two weeks before attempting to find them homes. When we put them up for adoption, Marshmellow found a home at the drop of a hat, but poor, sweet, little Cotton, — no one seemed to want a defective kitten.

I actually forget who came up with the Craig's List idea, but it was decided to place Cotton on Craig's List, clearly stating, so as to eliminate any misunderstandings, that the kitten had a congenital heart condition, and needed special care. Within thirty minutes after making the posting, a lady called and asked if Cotton was still available for adoption. Sandy told the caller that Cotton hadn't yet been adopted. The caller went on to say, "Oh good! My 16 year old daughter saw Cotton's posting, and immediately wanted her. You see, our daughter, Sara, also has a congenital heart defect. When she read the posting, her eyes lit up, and she told me that she felt a common bond with Cotton, — kind of a special, shared identity with the kitten. We'd sure like to adopt Cotton." Sandy asked the caller a few more questions, and then told her, "Sounds like Cotton has found herself the perfect home".

Sara and her mother were at the clinic bright and early the next day. It was truly heartwarming to see Sara embrace little Cotton, — they really were kindred spirits. I couldn't have imagined a better outcome for Cotton, and I was also happy for Sara. As the ole saying goes, "Ain't it great when a plan comes together".

sweet little "Cotton"

Oversexed Cat?

S eeing an animal for a "second opinion" was always an interesting and often delicate situation. The owners and their animals were clients and patients at other veterinary clinics or hospitals, and for whatever reason, the patient wasn't improving as expected. The owners had become increasingly frustrated at the lack of progress being made, and either questioned the original diagnosis, or simply needed reassurance that the diagnosis was correct and to stay on the course of treatment as prescribed.

Irma Walters, an eighty year old widow from a nearby town, had made an appointment to get a second opinion concerning a problem that her two year old cat, "Susie", was experiencing. Irma was on time for her appointment, and this very spry, white haired, diminutive senior citizen plopped the overweight grey tabby domestic shorthair cat on the exam table. I greeted the cat with, "Hi there Susie. What seems to be your problem?" Irma abruptly chimed in, "She's oversexed! That's what the other vet said, — just oversexed!" That statement caught me a little off guard. I'd never heard that one before, and I spontaneously blurted out, "Oversexed?" — "Yup, — that's what he said." Irma retorted. I immediately looked at Susie's medical records, and it stated right there in black and white that she was spayed. So I asked Irma, "It says on her records that she was spayed at six months of age. — Is that right?" Irma replied, "Yes, but she still comes into heat, — cries out with a strange sound, rolls all over the place, and raises her hind end up in the air. I took her back to the vet, and asked him if he took everything out. He said that he did, — but when I asked him why was she still coming back into heat, he just said that the cat was OVERSEXED! So, that's why I'm here, to get a second opinion, because that just didn't sound right to me." That didn't sound right to me either. "Mrs. Walters", I said, "Sometimes, — if a tiny bit of ovary were missed or re-tained during the surgical procedure, then that very small piece of ovary would be sufficient reproductive tissue to generate enough estrogen hormone to cause the cat to come into heat. If that is the case with Susie, then it could be very difficult to find that minus-cule piece of tissue in her abdomen, especially now that she has put on some extra pounds, and has a lot of fat on the inside. Irma responded, "Well, we've got to do something for the poor girl. She can't go on like this. It's hard on her, — and me too." I told Irma that I would schedule Susie for an exploratory surgery, and hopefully I'd find some retained ovarian tissue, remove it, and then the problem would be resolved.

The day for Susie's surgery had arrived, and she was anes-thetized, shaved, and prepped for the exploratory laparotomy. Susie was a pudgy little girl, and I knew that finding a remnant of ovarian tissue hiding in all that abdominal fat would be like finding a needle in a haystack. I made a longer incision in order to gain more exposure for the ensuing "treasure hunt". Wow! She had more than her share of fat in the abdominal cavity. The good thing was that her fat was whiter in color, which is usually the case with younger individuals. The whiter color would allow more contrast of any retained tissue. Nothing was found on the left side. However, on the right side, deep in the abdominal cav-ity, nestled within the white abdominal fat in the vicinity of where a normal ovary would be found, there was a small pink piece of tissue, about the size of the head of a stick pin, — about 2mm in diameter. That's what I was looking for! I excised the tissue, and felt confident that I'd found and removed the culprit. I then put Susie back together, and she recovered beautifully. The specimen was sent to the histology lab for microscopic identification, and several days later the lab report confirmed that it was indeed ovarian tissue, and that it had been completely excised.

I called Irma and when I told her the results of the lab report she said, "That's good news! I knew there had to be something causing the problem, and that there was more to it than just being oversexed." Susie was Irma's lap cat who remained portly, and never went into heat again. Oh yeah, the neighborhood tom cats stopped visiting her too. It was a real success story, and truly a big relief for both Irma and Susie.

Extreme Facial Makeover

A ndrea Kramer was a consummate librarian at a large high school in a nearby city. This very intelligent lady had a deep passion for cats, and took it upon herself to help any homeless cat that ventured her way. Andrea lived in an area of town that had more than its share of traffic, so it wasn't a surprise when she called about a cat that had just been hit by a car, — but at midnight!

It had been a busy, but productive day at the veterinary clinic. What I really needed now was a nice quiet evening at home and a good night's sleep. It was about 11:30 that night when the phone rang and roused me from my deep sleep. My first thought was, "Oh no, — an emergency! — Maybe it's a wrong number. — I sure hope so." I answered the phone with, "Dr. Roloff here.", and that's as far as I got before the caller interjected, "I'm sorry for calling you at home at this time of night. — Thank you for picking up. — This is Andrea. — Gretel just got hit by a car! — She looks bad! — I don't think she'll make it till morning. — Can I bring her in, – now?" I told Andrea to get Gretel in the car and I'd meet them at the clinic. I got up, dressed, grabbed a quick cup of coffee, and drove to the clinic with the car windows down to help clear the cobwebs.

It was about midnight when Andrea pulled up and walked through the clinic door with a severely injured cat named "Gretel" held gently in her arms. Gretel, a petite, black domestic shorthair, one of Andrea's personal favorites, looked to be in pretty tough shape and barely hanging on to life. Gretel had to be given I.V. medications immediately to counteract shock, and once stabilized, she could then be evaluated more thoroughly. Poor little Gretel's head was all messed up! She was struggling to breathe, and her face was physically distorted. Her right eye was protruding from the eye socket, and the pupil of her left eye was "pinpoint", very constricted, suggesting a concussion. Gretel's lower jaw was misaligned and unstable, likely fractured, and her hard palate (roof of the mouth) was split wide open, approximately 1 cm, providing a clear view directly inside her nasal cavity. Andrea asked, "Can you save her? Please say yes! She's such a good girl." I told Andrea, "It doesn't look good! For starters, Gretel has a concussion, and she'll be blind in her right eye because the optic nerve was damaged beyond repair when the eye was prolapsed (displaced from the socket). I'll try to replace the eye into the socket for esthetic purposes, but I can't guarantee anything. Her lower jaw is fractured at its mid-point, needs to be repositioned and stabilized with stainless steel surgical wire, and the gaping split of her hard palate needs to be sutured closed." I went on to tell Andrea I was quite concerned about Gretel having inhaled blood from the traumatized hard palate, and there was a distinct possibility of her developing pneumonia. Not a good thing!

Gretel was a surgical risk, but I had no recourse. Reconstructing the separated palate would be challenging, but I thought I could successfully pull it off. Gretel was anesthetized, blood was suctioned from her mouth and throat, and she was intubated. Positioning her head at the correct angle was critical in providing the best exposure to that tiny space. There wasn't a lot of room available to work, but in time, the delicate procedure was completed, and the split roof of her mouth was reunited. Next, Gretel's head was x-rayed to check for bone fractures, and her lower jaw (mandible) was the only fracture seen. The symphysis (the center union point of the right and left sides of the lower jaw bone) was broken and very unstable. Stainless steel surgical wire was used to realign and stabilize the jaw bone. Now she'd be able to eat. The final procedure involved replacing her protruding (prolapsed) right eye to its normal position. A canthotomy (incision at the outer corner of the eyelids) was made to create more space for ease of reducing (replacing) the prolapsed eye. The procedure was successful, but the eye would be blind because of the damage to the optic nerve. The only thing left to do was to clean and treat the superficial scrapes and minor cuts. I was done! Gretel was now back together, and she looked a whole lot better too! Gretel was a good patient and fortunate as well, because Andrea gave her excellent home care following all that reconstructive surgery. The roof of her mouth and jaw healed nicely, and the right eye, although blind, looked essentially normal.

Gretel had an unconquerable spirit, and was a very lucky little girl. She was blessed to have a loving owner like Andrea who was willing to do what was necessary to save her. Gretel had learned a valuable lesson about busy streets, was graced out, and went on to live a long and pampered life. You couldn't hope for anything better than that!

"Gretel"

About-Face

Preconceived notions can deprive an individual from experiencing some very enriching relationships. Such was the case with Fred Limpkin, a retired Air Force veteran. For some unknown reason Fred disliked cats, but he loved his dogs, and doted over his twenty-four year old Pekinese named, "Ming", until she passed on. Now, for the first time in many years, Fred was without an animal companion.

Fred's son, Mark, had recently graduated from college and accepted a job on the East coast. The cross-country move was a great career opportunity for Mark, but he couldn't take his big ebony colored cat, "Blackjack" along with him right away. So, Mark reluctantly asked his dad to care for Blackjack for a few months, knowing full well that Fred hated cats. Fred wasn't too keen about the idea, but eventually gave in, — but only after setting down some ground rules that included the cat staying out of his way!

Blackjack quickly settled into his "new digs", and seemed to take a particular liking to Fred. He started following Fred around the house like some groupie idolizing a rock star. Wherever Fred would go, — Blackjack was close behind. When Fred sat down in his favorite chair, the cat tried to join him, — only to be quickly and sternly rebuffed. Those two were the epitome of the "odd couple", — yet Blackjack's fondness for Fred never faltered. Gradually Fred became more tolerant of the cat's incessant need for contact, and eventually conceded, — and began gently stroking the big black cat that had finally made it onto his lap. Blackjack knew what he wanted, and sensed that in time, persistence would pay off, — and it did.

A bond between those two gradually developed and strengthened over the next few months. Fred had come to enjoy Blackjack's company, and even accompanied him to the vet clinic for exams and vaccinations. On one particular visit, Fred told me, "Ya know Doc, – here I am, almost seventy years old, and this is my first cat. I never knew how good a friend they could be. But this guy is really somthin special." He gently patted the big ebony cat several times, — smiled contentedly, — thoroughly smitten with the cat. He went on to say, with a certain tone of regret in his voice, "And to think that I used to hate cats. — I sure missed out on a lot for all those years." I reassured Fred, "Hey, — better late than never." It was a bit of a tense situation when Mark came back to visit and retrieve his black cat. Fred had become quite attached to Blackjack, and wasn't about to relinquish his "buddy". Mark saw the tight bond that'd been forged between those two, and wisely chose not to rock the boat, and let them remain together.

It was truly uplifting to witness the joy that those two brought to each other. As the years passed, both aged gracefully, but then Fred, unfortunately, was diagnosed with having terminal cancer. During those ensuing months of illness, Blackjack never left Fred's side, and was a constant source of comfort and companionship through the hard times. Then one day Mrs. Limpkin phoned the clinic and said that Blackjack, now sixteen years old, was vomiting and not eating. An appointment was scheduled, and when the time had arrived, — a pale, feeble, very sick old man came shuffling through the front door of the clinic, with a black cat gently cradled in his arms. Fred, as ill as he was, was not about to abandon his "buddy" in time of need. One quick glance at this man, and it was glaringly apparent that he didn't have much time left on this earth! Blackjack was thin, weak, listless, dehydrated, vomiting, anorexic, and had that strong, foul, ketone odor on his breath. — all signs associated with kidney failure! Blood tests were needed for confirmation, and the results left no doubt whatsoever, —— Blackjack indeed was in the final stages of kidney failure, — and he wasn't going to make it much longer. I spoke to Mrs. Limpkin in another room, and delivered the bad news. She asked, "Can you keep him going a week or two? I don't want him to die before Fred does. — He really needs that cat." I assured Mrs. Limpkin that I'd do my best to keep Blackjack alive and comfortable for as long as possible. — and I did. Blackjack was placed on I.V. fluids initially, given subcutaneous fluids and special nutritional supplementation daily, and also received medications to calm the nausea, and vomiting. His condition stabilized, he was relatively comfortable, and wasn't suffering. We'd achieved our goal.

Fred died the following week with Blackjack by his side, and Blackjack departed to be with Fred just a few days later. That ebony colored cat had changed Fred's attitude about cats from downright distain to absolute affection. — He'd undergone an amazing "About-Face". Blackjack enabled Fred to experience the joy, comfort, and companionship of a loving cat, — and those two remained faithful friends and buddies to the very end.

A Triple Whammy

We've all heard the expression, "Things happen in threes", and most of us have experienced this uncanny phenomenon. Is it just a coincidence, or is it some kind of self-fulfilling prophecy? We'll never know, but one thing is sure, —— it does happen.

Mandy Ann was one of the happiest dogs I'd ever seen. Nothing seemed to ever bother this ten year old Springer Spaniel. She was unflappable, and had that Alfred E. Newman philosophy of life, — "What? Me worry?". She loved to come to the vet clinic because she knew she'd get goodies from the "treat man", — me. I'll admit that maybe I'd give her a few extra treats during her clinic visits, — but hey, we were having fun, and I enjoyed spoiling her, — just a little bit.

Mandy Ann's owner, Karen Jones, had become concerned about a bulge that was growing on the inside of Mandy Ann's lower right eyelid, and she wanted it "checked out". When Mandy Ann arrived at the clinic, she ran straight into the exam room and promptly sat directly in front of HER "treat" drawer. She wasn't bothered by the fact that another dog was on the table and I was in the middle of an examination. Karen sternly yelled out from the waiting room, "Mandy Ann, you come back here right now! It isn't your turn yet." Mandy Ann reluctantly obeyed her owner's command, and left the room. Finally it was Mandy Ann's turn, and she jumped onto the lift table, anticipating the ride upward to my eye level. Her problem was staring me right in the face. — A large growth on the inside of her lower right eyelid, causing the eyelid to evert. The growth was firm, non-pigmented, and had been growing "pretty fast", according to the owner. Not good, because cancerous growths usually grow quite rapidly. I told Karen my concerns, and scheduled Mandy Ann for surgery ASAP. The surgery went well, and when Mandy Ann awoke from the anesthesia, she pranced out the clinic door as if nothing had happened. What a trooper! I sent the tumor to the histopathology lab for analysis, and was not surprised by the report. It was diagnosed as an amelanotic melanoma of the conjunctiva of the eyelid. The prognosis (outcome) was considered guarded (very serious), but the one bit of good news was that the tumor had been completely excised, and hopefully hadn't yet metastasized to the lymph nodes. Time would tell. Mandy Ann healed well and there were no complications.

About six months later Karen called the clinic and said, "Mandy Ann has been having some trouble eating, and moves her tongue around in a funny way. I opened her mouth and it looks like there is something growing under her tongue". Once again, Mandy Ann came bounding into the clinic as if she didn't have a care in the world. Upon opening her mouth, I could see a tumor about the size of a large egg growing on the right side of her tongue, and it was pushing her tongue to the left. The tumor definitely had to be removed, but that also meant removing part of her tongue in the process. The tongue is a very vascular structure, and controlling the hemorrhage during surgery would undoubtedly be a challenge. Mandy Ann was scheduled for surgery, and once again she was an ideal patient. The surgical procedure went well, the amount of blood loss was marginal, but about one quarter of her tongue had to be removed. The histology report stated that the tumor was a squamous cell carcinoma, a potentially aggressive cancer that tends to invade the lymphatics and metastasizes to the lymph nodes. But the good news was that I'd had gotten it all out, even though the margins were small. Mandy Ann had once again dodged a bullet. That was her second major cancer surgery, and hopefully the last.

A year had passed, Mandy Ann's tongue had healed nicely and was functioning well, even with a good sized divot on the right side, — and her lower right eyelid looked as good as new with no regrowth of the tumor. However, — NOW, — Mandy Ann's LEFT upper eyelid was swollen. At first Karen thought it was a mosquito bite, and surmised that she'd just wait for it to go away, — but it never did. When I examined the "swelling", it felt hard and appeared to be growing WITHIN the eyelid itself. This was Mandy Ann's THIRD tumor within a relatively short period of time. The tumorous growth could not be easily accessed from the underside of the eyelid, only from the top, outer surface. The problem with removing the tumor from the outer surface of the eyelid was the potential for cutting and/or damaging critical nerves to the eyelid itself. If that were to happen, she could end up with a permanently drooping upper eyelid. I consulted with eye and surgical specialists, and they weren't very encouraging. I told Karen the bad news and she asked, "Would you do the surgery? That's okay if she has a droopy eyelid, — I just don't want to do nothing, and watch her suffer." I took a deep breath and said, "All right, — I'll do the surgery, — but please understand that the outcome might be less than desired." Karen responded, "Oh Doc, I understand. — I'm just glad that you're willing to do it."

The surgery day for Mandy Ann had arrived, she was anesthetized, prepped, and positioned. It was a long, tedious, and delicate surgery. The tumor was firmly embedded within the tissue of the upper eyelid, and had to be painstakingly dissected free. Once removed, it was a tricky procedure to reconstruct the eyelid and close the empty cavity created by the tumor's absence, — but eventually I got it done. When Mandy Ann awoke, she was her old happy self, but with a swollen, bruised, and droopy eyelid. The histology report confirmed my suspicions. It was another amelanotic melanoma, and it had been completely excised. That was really good news! Mandy Ann made a successful recovery, and in time, as the swelling subsided, the eyelid still drooped, but much less than expected. — In fact, she held the eyelid three quarters of the way open most of the time, — kind of a modified wink. Karen was pleased.

Mandy Ann went on to live many more happy, tumor free years. She'd beaten three malignant tumor episodes within a relatively short period of time, and had none thereafter. So, there just might be something to that ole saying that, "Things happen in threes", or perhaps it could be said that, "The third time's the charm".

Getting Stoned!

B ob Dylan's songs and lyrics about getting "stoned" referred to layin back, chillin out, getting high, and having a good time. To my patients, getting stones or stoned meant that they couldn't pee, — and it wasn't fun! It was a painful and potentially life threatening experience for them.

Bladder stones, also referred to as uroliths or calculi, are solid masses or concretions of minerals, usually calcium, magnesium, or urates. They tend to form in the urinary bladder following a bacterial infection in the urinary tract. The bladder stones can vary in size, shape, and color, depending upon their mineral content, and the number of stones present can also range from just a single stone to many of different sizes. Smaller ones, about the size of a BB or smaller, often pass easily, especially with females, because they have bigger plumbing. Larger stones, however, usually restrict or totally obstruct urine flow, and that could lead to a life threatening situation. In most cases, surgical intervention with the removal of the bladder stones, is the only viable solution to the problem.

"Coco"

Angela, our receptionist, answered the phone, talked briefly to the caller, then turned to me and said, "You need to talk to this lady, Doc. She wants you to GIVE her antibiotics for her dog's bladder infection, — but doesn't want the dog examined. We've never seen animals for this person, — she's new to the area." I took the phone, introduced myself, and asked, "What seems to be the problem with your dog?" The caller, Ms. Myrna Krume, sternly replied, "My dog has a bladder or urine infection and is leaking urine all the time! I've seen this before because I've raised a lot of dogs. — All she needs is some antibiotics." I told Ms. Krume, "Your dog really needs to be examined because there are other conditions, in addition to bacterial infections that can cause your dog to leak urine. She could have bladder stones, tumors, or even a hormone imbalance problem. I can't just hand out antibiotics indiscriminately." Ms. Krume was not particularly happy, and told me that her other vet would have given her the antibiotics. I responded by telling Ms. Krume that I was NOT her other vet, and that I wouldn't compromise! Ms. Krume mumbled a few unintelligible words, but then reluctantly made an appointment for the dog to be seen.

Ms. Krume was on time for the appointment, and plopped the miniature poodle, named "Coco", on the exam table. Coco was a sweet, but timid, chocolate colored little girl. As I palpated (felt) her urinary bladder, I detected a large, solid structure that seemed to occupy the entire bladder. I told Ms. Krume that I suspected a large urolith was causing the problem, and I needed to take an x-ray for confirmation, and also check for any smaller stones. Ms. Krume looked at me with a skeptical expression, told me that she'd never heard of such a thing in dogs, but eventually gave her consent, —grudgingly. Coco was a good patient, and laid quietly while the x-ray was taken. The developed x-ray revealed a HUGE, solitary stone about the size of an extra, extra large egg. It literally took up all the interior space of the urinary bladder, leaving absolutely no room for the urine to accumulate. The urine essentially flowed around the gigantic stone, then leaked out. No wonder Coco was leaking urine almost constantly. — It couldn't be held in the bladder, — no room!!! I showed the x-ray to Ms.

Krume, who wasn't overly impressed, and told her that Coco needed to have the urolith surgically removed immediately. Ms. Krume once again mumbled a few words under her breath, but finally conceded that the surgery was necessary.

The surgery went well. An abdominal incision was made, the urinary bladder was then incised, and the humongous bladder stone was successfully removed. Coco was put back together, re-covered nicely, and was maintained on I.V. fluids and antibiotics for the next twenty-four hours. All systems were working as they should, and "amazingly", — Coco wasn't dribbling urine any-more! Wow! Go figure! I showed the huge bladder stone, which incidentally had conformed to the exact shape of the bladder, to Ms. Krume, but she was UNDERwhelmed, and didn't say a word.

That would be the first, — and the last time I'd ever see Ms. Krume and Coco. For whatever reason, Ms. Krume never re-turned. One thing to feel good about was the fact that I'd relieved the pain and suffering of a sweet, and very forgiving little dog, made her much more comfortable, and essentially saved her life.

"Abby"

Christmas Eve is a special time for getting together with fam-ily and friends, attending church services, and phoning loved ones with season's greetings. It was 7:30 P.M. on one particular Christmas Eve when the telephone rang. Sandy quickly grabbed the phone, anticipating a call from our son. It wasn't him. — it was Jerry Pratter.

"I'm sorry for calling you on Christmas Eve, but I don't know what else to do. It's Abby, — She's very sick and really weak. I don't think she's going to make it. Could you please take a look at her?" Sandy handed me the phone and said, "We've got an emer-gency!" My heart sunk. All my plans for the evening went right out the window. —A patient and her owner desperately needed help, and that took precedence! I dropped what I was doing and told Jerry to bring Abby to the clinic right away.

Sandy and I rushed to the vet clinic and began preparing for the emergency. A few minutes later Mr. Pratter entered the clinic clutching a limp, seemingly lifeless little white dog in his arms. Jerry and his wife Dawn again apologized for interrupting our Christmas Eve, and graciously thanked us for being there to help. Abby, a young Bichon Frise, was extremely weak, had pale mucous membranes, diminished reflexes, and her heart rate and respirations were alarmingly slow. Her abdomen was tender and her urinary bladder was grossly distended. A quick x-ray showed a small bladder stone lodged in the urethrae, preventing any urine from exiting the bladder. I inserted a long needle through the skin and into the bladder, removed 40cc of urine, which temporarily decreased the distention and eased some of the pain. Abby's condition was rapidly deteriorating, — she was on her way out, — and she'd surely die if that bladder stone wasn't removed IMMEDIATELY, —— NOW!!! We didn't have much time! It was definitely a life-or-death situation. I explained Abby's critical condition to the Pratters, and the possibility of her not making it through the surgery. They understood the surgical risks, and were willing to take the chance.

The surgical procedure was very challenging, — to say the least! The urinary bladder was incised and a small forceps was inserted in the bladder, then through the neck of the bladder, and finally into the urethrae. A small, bean-shaped, tightly wedged bladder stone was then grasped with the tip of the forceps, gently maneuvered free, and removed. Urine started flowing immediately, — like gangbusters! — problem solved!!!

Abby made it through the surgery, although there were several moments where things got pretty "Touch-n-Go", — but that tough little gal hung in there! She did good!! Jerry and Dawn were overjoyed and understandably very thankful that Abby had pulled through. Believe me, that was one Christmas Eve they'll never forget, —— and neither will I!

"Abby" fully recovered.

"Bruce"

Bruce wasn't your typical farm dog. He was a pudgy, well groomed, purebred miniature Schnauzer who loved pickups and country life. He was his owner's little sidekick.

Wayne Steppe, Bruce's owner, had become concerned about his little buddy's recent behavior. Mr. Steppe said, "Bruce acts like he's trying to, "go", — and nothing comes out except a few drops. He just stands there with his legs spread and back hunched up, but nothing happens. He acts like something's plugged up." I told Wayne that it sure sounded that way, and a couple x-rays should give us some answers. The x-rays showed that Bruce wasn't con-stipated, and there weren't any blockages in the urinary bladder, — BUT there was a small bladder stone that had moved from the bladder, down through the urethrae, and was now lodged behind the os penis (a bony structure in the male dog's penis through which the urethrae passes). That bony structure doesn't allow the urethrae to expand, so a small stone lodged behind the os penis would definitely stop the flow of urine. Bruce was in major trou-ble, — he couldn't pee,— and he needed help, — PRONTO!

The small urolith (calculi), a little larger than a bb, could not be pushed retrograde (backward) into the urinary bladder, nor could it move forward through the os penis. My only option was to surgically remove the calculi through a ventral (underside) inci-sion through the skin, subcutaneous tissue and then the extremely thin urethrae. After removing the small stone, I reconstructed a new, larger and permanent underneath opening for Bruce.

The surgery was a very delicate procedure, but a complete suc-cess, and Bruce didn't have to strain to void anymore. It did look a little unusual though, because whenever Bruce felt the urge, he'd hike his leg to pee, and urine passed out the "NEW" porthole on the underside of his penis. It may have looked a little weird, — but he didn't seem to mind.

Foreign Bodies

Life can get awfully complicated when things are out of order or in places they shouldn't be. That scenario was often seen when animals ingested objects other than food, and when that happened, those "foreign bodies" usually created some very big problems.

"Domino"

"Domino", a two year old black and white domestic short-hair cat, with a voracious appetite, had recently refused to eat his food. That concerned his owner, Sally Ahern. She told Heather, our veterinary technician, "Domino is usually a very lively and playful cat, but now he just sits in the corner, — all hunched up in the middle, and doesn't want to move." Mrs. Ahern didn't want something bad to happen to her young daughter's special friend, so she made an appointment to have Domino checked over.

Domino was a very docile cat who didn't object to being examined. His temperature was normal, he was moderately dehydrated, but when I felt his abdomen — he flinched and pulled away — BINGO! I told Mrs. Ahern that Domino was very painful in the upper abdominal area, and x-rays might show us why. The x-rays revealed a dense, oddly shaped, foreign object seemingly trapped in his stomach, — and it didn't belong there! — The handwriting was on the wall. — Surgery!

Domino was quickly prepped for surgery, — and in we went. A gastrotomy (incising the stomach) procedure can be tricky, and extra caution is required to avoid spilling contaminated stomach contents into the abdominal cavity. The surgery on Domino went flawlessly. — The stomach was incised, nothing spilled, the mysterious invader was isolated, grasped with a forceps, removed, and placed in a tray for further examining. I told him, "Hey Domino little buddy, you should be a lot more comfortable now with that thing outa there. I closed, placed him in the recovery cage, and we were done.

The mysterious object turned out to be a small, wooden, rubber stamp with an image of a cartoon character on it. When I showed Mrs. Ahern the object that was removed, she exclaimed, "Oh my gosh! — That's one of my daughter's favorite toys. — She plays with them all the time. I've seen Domino batting those little stamps around the house, and he likes carrying them in his mouth too. I never thought that he'd actually eat or swallow one of them." I advised Mrs. Ahern to go home and pick up all the small toys and tiny objects so that Domino isn't tempted to become a repeat offender.

Domino went on to make a complete recovery, — and all those little wooden stamps amazingly disappeared from her daughter's toy box.

"Bobby"

Phil Stangley called the clinic and told our receptionist that he was worried about his ten week old Springer Spaniel named Bobby, and then he said, "The last couple days, when he tries to poop, — he squats, strains a little, — then cries. — Then he turns around and licks his butt."

Bobby was a cute little guy, specially with those long brown ears. He didn't look sick, in fact he acted like a normal puppy when first placed on the exam table, but cried when he sat down. As I raised his tail to examine the rectal area, Bobby whimpered again. I noticed a "tenting" of skin just slightly to the left of the rectum, as if something was embedded and poking from under the skin. When palpated, it felt hard and pointed. X-rays were taken, and I was amazed at what appeared on the films. It was a two inch sewing needle! I placed a local anesthetic at the "tenting" site, made a very small, 1/4 inch incision, and like magic, the pointed tip of the needle popped into view. Using a small forceps, I grasped the needle and applied slow, gentle and steady retraction. The needle was easily withdrawn, but I was surprised to see that there was at least 12 inches of heavyweight thread still attached to the needle. The surgical site was then medicated, and only one suture (stitch) was needed to close the small incision.

Bobby healed very nicely without any complications. The odds were extremely small for a swallowed needle and thread to successfully pass down the esophagus, into and through the stomach, then on through the tortuous small and large intestines, — and almost make it out the rectum. The needle could have punctured or penetrated the viscera, and the thread could have become entangled, both of which might have been life threatening to little Bobby. It was nothing short of a miracle for everything to almost pass completely through like it did.

I kept the needle and thread in a special formalin specimen bottle as a teaching aid. Clients could see, first hand, what needs to be kept away from inquisitive puppies. Phil also made sure that his wife was more careful with her sewing stuff.

"Jerry"

Jerry was a three year old German Shepard who was having digestive problems for several weeks. His owner, Mary Farmer, tried to help Jerry by offering him a bland diet consisting of boiled hamburger and rice. She also gave him a kaopectate tablet twice a day in an attempt to firm up his soft, unformed stools. Jerry's condition hadn't improved, so Mrs. Farmer made an appointment to have him examined, treated, and put back to normal, —— at minimal expense.

When I examined Jerry, he appeared to be under weight, almost malnourished. His coat was dry and dull, and he lacked energy and enthusiasm. — He was pretty blah. His rectal temperature was normal, but he winced and pulled away in discomfort when I palpated his abdomen. There was a section of the small intestine that felt larger than normal, somewhat thickened, and that concerned me. "Mrs. Farmer", I said. "I think Jerry might have an intestinal obstruction." Mrs. Farmer couldn't understand how that could happen. She went on to say, "Jerry is always with me, and I watch what he eats, so I don't see how he could have eaten anything to cause this. I don't give him bones or anything that's hard to digest." I went on to explain about other conditions such as intussusceptions (telescoping) of the intestines, and malabsorption conditions that could exhibit similar signs. I told Mrs. Farmer that a stool analysis, blood tests, and x-rays were highly recommended and needed in order to get to the bottom of Jerry's problem. Mrs. Farmer declined the tests and x-rays, — and was essentially looking for an "easy fix". I thought I'd ask just one more question. "Mrs. Farmer, could Jerry have ingested any of his toys or some child's toy?" She emphatically replied, "No! He doesn't eat his toys, and he hasn't been around any kids either." So, — getting nowhere, — I placed Jerry on gastrointestinal sedatives, G.I. protectants, and a special diet specific for diarrheas and malabsorption conditions. I firmly told Mrs. Farmer that if Jerry didn't improve in one week, then x-rays MUST be taken. Mrs. Farmer nodded her head in agreement.

A week passed, and Jerry hadn't improved, in fact his condition had worsened. Mrs. Farmer finally conceded that x-rays were necessary. The x-ray films revealed a strange semi-transparent object wedged in the small intestine and surgical removal was the only recourse. Jerry was prepped, and into surgery we went. I made an abdominal incision, and the swollen, inflamed, and discolored section of small intestine wasn't difficult to isolate. The small intestine was carefully incised open (enterotomy), and the offending object was gently removed with the aid of a forceps. As I dropped the object into the tray held by my surgical assistant, I said, "Here,—— have a baby bottle nipple!" Jerry was put back together, transferred to the recovery room, and was maintained on I.V. fluids for the next 24 hours. He recovered nicely.

I showed the rubber baby bottle nipple, which also had the end chewed off, to Mrs. Farmer. She was surprised, and said, "Oh, I forgot. Jerry had been over to my daughter's house, and he must have gotten ahold of her baby's bottle." Finally the pieces of the puzzle had come together, and the mystery was solved!

Jerry made a dramatically successful recovery. He started eating again, gained weight, had normal stools, and developed a nice shiny hair coat. He looked like any other healthy German Shepard now, — minus the baby bottle nipple that was wedged in his gut!!!

"Mac"

Some dogs are fiercely independent, and hate to be shackled by a collar, no matter what it looks like. "Mac", a Pitt Bull cross, was one of those dogs. He'd destroyed his share of collars, but when his owner, Paul Verdel, found a super heavy-duty, double reinforced, one inch wide collar, he thought, "there's no way Mac will get this thing off".

It wasn't but a few days, and the collar was off. Mac had shown Paul who was boss. The only problem, —— Paul couldn't find the collar! Oh sure, he found a few pieces, but the bulk of the collar was missing. Paul thought that Mac might have buried it somewhere around the yard, but couldn't find any evidence.

It wasn't but a few days later that a listless Mac started vomiting, and Paul entertained the notion that Mac could have actually eaten the dang thing. Paul brought his sick buddy to the clinic, told me the history, and asked if there was anything that could be done for Mac. I told Paul, "First, — I start with x-rays to check for any possible abnormalities in the digestive tract." The x-ray films showed several areas where the intestines appeared to be bunched up together. — Not a good sign! Paul asked, "If the collar is in there, can you get it out? I'd sure hate to lose ole Mac." I told Paul that I'd do the best I could to help Mac, but sometimes with obstructions, there can be irreparable damage to the intestinal tissue, — some can be saved, — some can't.

Mac's surgery was a long and painstaking procedure. He had indeed eaten the collar. There where seven separate sections of the chewed-up collar, connected by several strands of nylon fiber, and those sections were dispersed throughout Mac's intestines. So, seven separate enterotomies (incisions into the intestine) were needed to completely remove the collar. One enterotomy operation is bad enough, but to do seven on the same patient was unbelievable. It was touch-n-go for Mac, but he made it through the surgery. Now, time would tell if the tissue was viable, and if the intestinal sutures held. Any leakage of intestinal contents into the abdominal cavity would have been disastrous. Mac was kept on intravenous fluids for two days, plus antibiotics and a soft bland diet for ten days. He was a pretty sore boy for a while, but he made a slow and steady recovery back to his normal self. Mac was fortunate to have survived the ordeal. Paul also learned a valuable lesson, and from that time on, he still let Mac run free, — but without a collar.

"Other Cases"

Over the years, I surgically removed many different kinds of foreign bodies from both cats and dogs. In addition to those already mentioned, the "Hall of the De-famed" included hazelnuts, rocks, glass fragments, a cigarette lighter with lighter fluid still inside, balls, fishing lures, socks, and small toys. Fortunately, all my surgical patients survived their ordeal, and hopefully learned from their experience.

It Was Meant to Be

Some of the most endearing creatures on the face of the earth are healthy puppies and kittens. These cute little bundles of energy bring joy to our lives, and shower us with unconditional love. Their playful antics make us laugh, and give us momentary stress relief from the hectic events we deal with every day. These precious little ones are truly gifts from God.

Tiger, an eight week old brown classic tabby, was a very special kitten. His owner, Penny Tatem, carried him under her light jacket into the exam room for his first vaccinations. When Penny handed Tiger to me, he immediately positioned himself under my chin and then began to purr. He sought security in close, intimate contact. This gentle and affectionate kitten was a real charmer.

It had been over a year since I'd last seen Tiger. In most cases, no news is good news, but not in this instance. Penny called the clinic, and with a voice filled with anxiety, she told our receptionist, "I'm a little concerned about Tiger. He just hasn't been himself lately. He doesn't act especially painful, but somethings definitely not right and I think he needs to be seen by the doctor." When Tiger arrived at the clinic, I was a little surprised to see how big and handsome he'd become. He sat nonchalantly on the exam table, almost oblivious to all the activity going on around him. He was stoically preoccupied with discomfort of some nature, and now it was up to me to find the source of the problem. As I palpated his abdomen, an enlarged section of his intestines could easily be felt. He was, without question, uncomfortable, and x-rays would be needed to help clarify what was going on inside his little body. Penny's finances were limited, and she expressed that she couldn't afford, — nor was she interested in treating Tiger. She bluntly said with an obvious lack of emotion, "Just put him down!" I was caught off guard, to say the least. As I looked into Tiger's big amber colored eyes, I recalled the gentle little kitten that once cuddled under my chin. I wanted to help him, not "deep six" him. So, I asked Penny if she'd consider relinquishing ownership of Tiger to me, I'd do the workups and surgery, if needed, and that way he might have a chance to live. Without a moment's hesitation, Penny signed the transfer of ownership papers, and now Tiger was legally mine. Saving his life was priority number one.

X-rays were quickly taken of Tiger's abdomen, and the developed films revealed a huge problem. There appeared to be a six inch section of Tiger's small intestine that was obstructed with something that couldn't be easily identified. It really didn't matter at that point, because whatever it was, it had to be removed, —— IMMEDIATELY! Tiger was anesthetized, prepped, IV catheter placed, and within minutes I made the initial abdominal incision. The problem section of small intestine was quickly and easily identified because of its increased size and discoloration. I carefully isolated and packed off the surgical site to avoid any contamination of intestinal contents into the abdominal cavity, and then proceeded to perform an enterotomy, (incising open the intestines). There it was! A large, long wad of twisted, entangled dried decorator plant material that Tiger had obviously eaten. I delicately removed the offending obstruction, then surgically closed the intestinal and abdominal incisions. Tiger was administered antibiotics, and while still hooked up to fluids, he was placed in a nice warm recovery cage. I'd done all that I could do, and it was now up to Tiger. When He awoke from the anesthesia, he stood up, stretched, and started meowing for food and attention. It was truly astounding!!! He acted as if nothing had happened!

Sandy had a greeting card with a beautiful charcoal sketch of a big cat reclining in a wicker basket on the front of the card. It was entitled, "Henry's Basket". Amazingly, that cat looked almost exactly like Tiger! Now that Tiger belonged to us, and he'd gotten a new lease on life, Sandy thought he also deserved a new name. So, — we named him, —— "HENRY"!

Henry has been part of our family for twelve years. He is one of the most gentle, affectionate, and intuitive cats that I have ever seen. Henry has been my constant companion who loves to be with me and held,—— and yes, that svelte 15 pound cat still cuddles real close, with his head under my chin. Henry's a good boy. It's funny how life works, — how we found each other. It often seems like we were destined to be together. — I guess it was simply, — meant to be.

Doc Jim and "Henry"

Casanova Louie

The television action series, "MacGyver" ran from 1985 to 1992, and was a huge hit with the viewing public. The main character, named MacGyver, found himself in unusual dilemmas where he had to use his imagination to solve a problem. He was a very resourceful individual whose ingenuity allowed him to create unorthodox solutions to the challenges he encountered. Essentially he had to use his head and what was immediately available to make something work. Thus, the term, "MacGyvering" was coined, referring to the process of taking what was available, and successfully making it work. Over the years, there were occasions when I was confronted with a tough case that required some surgical "MacGyvering", and Louie was one of those cases.

Hazel Roemer was a respected and successful dog breeder of Miniature French Poodles. She had shown the dogs competitively, and her kennels had garnered many champions over the years. As time passed, her days of showing dogs was but a memory, however, this strong willed, seventy-eight year old woman still operated a breeding kennels in spite of her issues of being very arthritic and experiencing dwindling eyesight.

Hazel presented "King Louis of Avalon" a seven year old silver male French Poodle, one of her remaining breeding males, to the clinic because of a "licking" problem. Hazel told me, "Louie is constantly licking himself. I've looked, and I can't really see anything, but I can smell it, and it smells like he's got an infection." She went on to say, "It's getting harder for me to keep up with those dogs,—— I just can't get around like I used to, and I have trouble seeing these days." While Hazel was still talking, Louie got himself into a comfortable sitting position, and started licking at his genital area again. I moved his head to the side so that I could get a better look, and saw the reason for his incessant licking, — and the foul smell. Half of his penis was black as coal, — necrotic, — rotten, — essentially gangrenous. "Hazel, here's why Louie's been licking so much and smells so bad," I said. "His penis is rotting off." Hazel bent over and got close enough to see for herself. She then asked, "How could this have happened?" I told her that it was hard to tell, but something had clearly interfered with the circulation of blood to the area, because there was such a well defined line of distinction between the healthy tissue and the necrotic tissue. I could tell by Hazel's facial expressions and demeanor that she really cared for little Louie, and was very concerned about him. She soberly asked, "Can anything be done for my poor Louie?" I told her that Louie couldn't live this way, and there was no other choice but to amputate his penis, reconstruct a new opening for him to pee through, and also neuter him. Hazel was more than willing to have the surgical procedure done for her favorite little poodle, especially if it meant possibly saving his life.

Louie was anesthetized, prepped, and it was now time to do some major surgical "MacGyvering". I amputated the necrotic penis, removed the os penis (bony structure), and performed a urethrostomy. A urethrostomy is a procedure that creates a new permanent opening of the urethra to the exterior, and this new opening allows for the passing of urine. After that was successfully completed, I then neutered him. He had gotten the "Full Monty". Louie had gone from the main breeder in Hazel's kennel to a little guy who literally didn't have any equipment remaining. His breeding days were definitely over, but he was alive and could live a good life, and that's what really mattered. Following the surgery, I dissected the amputated penis, looking for a possible cause for the problem. I found a cord-like band of twisted hair that had somehow gotten up inside the sheath of the penis and wrapped itself around the base of the penis,—— effectively strangulating the feeder vessels, and that ultimately resulted in the death of the tissue (necrosis). The mystery was solved!

Louie made a rapid recovery, his new pee-port was working as it should, he stopped licking at his genitals, and once again, he acted like a "normal" dog. Hazel was quite pleased, but two weeks later she called the clinic and had a question for me. "Doctor Roloff, Louie is doing very well, but I thought you said that you neutered him. He sure doesn't act like he's been neutered. He's out there mounting all the females that are coming into heat, and he acts like the Romeo he'd always been. I assured Hazel that all his male parts were gone,— they were history, — he had nada. I was glad to hear that Louie was back to his ole self, and told her, "It's like the saying goes, "Old habits die hard", and Casanova Louie is livin' in the past, except now he's just shootin blanks."

Animal Crackers

We've all had experiences that have left indelible images etched in our minds. Some of those images are pleasant, some aren't, and no matter how hard we try, we just can't erase them from our psyche. The "Frankie incident" was one of those unpleasant experiences that created a repulsive mental picture which has endured in my mind for years.

Frankie was a five year old Dachshund who was the canine version of Dennis-the-menace. He was a mischievous little guy who kept his owner on her toes, so it came as no surprise when he helped himself to a large bag of frosted animal crackers. Frankie definitely had too much of a good thing, and was now reaping the consequences. His swollen abdomen, and lack of energy prompted his owner, Sue Milton, to rush him to the clinic for help.

When Frankie arrived at the clinic, he was really hurtin'. His abdomen was grossly distended, and that boy was really uncomfortable. He just stood there on the exam table with his legs slightly splayed and his neck extended forward in an attempt to ease some of the abdominal pain. It was imperative to get all that stuff out of his stomach, — and that meant making him vomit. I immediately went to the emergency crash cart, grabbed the apomorphine, placed a small amount into the conjunctival space of his left eye, and within thirty seconds, Frankie pitched it! — He lost his cookies, — literally! I let him retch and vomit several more times to ensure complete emptying of the stomach before rinsing out his eye with saline solution, in an attempt to remove any residual apomorphine and stop the induced vomiting. Once the purging episode was over with, Frankie just stood there, much relieved, and definitely more comfortable! His abdomen had returned to its normal size, and he looked around as if to say, "What the heck just happened?" — I can tell you what just happened. There on the exam table was a large, foul-smelling, pool of vomit, — consisting of mushed up, partially digested animal crackers, with swirls of pink and white frosting everywhere. There were also hundreds of those tiny round blue and white candy sprinkles floating all throughout the whole stinking mess. It was gross and disgusting, but Frankie felt better, and that's what counted.

Frankie left the clinic acting as if nothing had happened. He bounded out the door, bright-eyed and bushy-tailed, — looking for his next misadventure. I cautioned his owner to be very watchful and keep all cookies out of Frankie's reach, but we both knew that would be a major challenge. Frankie was a lovable little guy who was, and remained to be, an accident waiting to happen. To say that Frankie had a profound effect on me, would be a complete and total understatement. To this very day, I cannot look at an animal cracker, especially those pink and white frosted ones, without recalling little Frankie, and visualizing the vomit scene on the exam table. That mental image is permanently etched in my memory bank, and has forever curbed my appetite for animal crackers.

Road Warrior

It's never a pretty scene when cars and animals cross paths. Some animals miraculously escape the carnage, while others may survive, but they pay a high price with broken bodies and permanent scars. Then there are those who never get a second chance. It's always sad to see a deceased animal laying on the road, and there have been times when I've stopped and moved an animal's remains to the side of the road in an attempt to prevent any further desecration.

That particular day started out pretty uneventfully, but then the clinic door abruptly swung open and a lady stuck her head inside the door and blurted out, "I don't know who to tell, but there's a cat laying in the middle of the street just a block from here, and I think its dead.—— Somebody needs to pick it up and get it off the road so cars won't run over it." Although I was in the back of the clinic, I could definitely hear the lady, so I quickly went to the waiting room and assured her that I'd go immediately and take care of the situation. I grabbed a cadaver bag and latex gloves in preparation for the gruesome task, then jumped into the car, and was at the scene in very short order. She was right! Laying there all stretched out and motionless, smack dab in the middle of the street, was a younger looking black and white cat. I approached the cat, didn't see any blood, then checked its eyes and saw that the pupils were not yet fully dilated, — that was a hopeful sign. The cat, however, didn't appear to be breathing, but when I listened to the chest with my stethoscope, I heard a faint, slow heartbeat. I muttered to myself, "This cat is alive, — but barely!" Without delay, right there in the middle of the street, I started administering heart and chest compressions. That went on for about a minute or so when suddenly the cat's chest heaved, and it took a deep breath. YAHOO!!!! I continued the cardiac massage and chest compressions for a little while longer and then took another listen to the chest. The heartbeat sounded stronger and more regular, and the lung sounds were slightly raspy, but at least it was now breathing on its own. This cat had a good chance of making it, barring any major internal injuries or broken bones. I placed the recumbent cat ON the bag, instead of in it, and then rushed the patient back to the clinic.

I entered the clinic through the back door with the injured cat securely held in my arms, — and called out to the staff, "We've got a live one here! — I need some help! — get the oxygen and IV's ready!" Everyone immediately swung into emergency mode. — The cat was quickly hooked up to the oxygen. — I.V. catheters were placed. — Fluids started flowing into its veins, — and drugs to counter shock and tissue swelling were injected into the I.V. line. It was amazing and encouraging to see how fast the cat responded to the treatments. Once the cat was stabilized, we then started checking it over for other injuries, and in the process we found it to be a young male, about five months old, with a blue collar, — suggesting that he probably belonged to someone, and he had multiple scrapes, abrasions, and minor cuts, — typical "road rash" stuff. The injury of most concern, however, was the instability and grinding that was detected on the right side of his pelvis. X-rays were taken and showed that the little guy had a fracture at the midpoint of the body of the right ilium bone of the pelvis. It was a major break that resulted from the impact of the car. The repair options for fractures of that nature included surgical plating, wiring the pieces into place, or placement of an intramedullary (within the bone marrow) stainless steel rod (pin), either by open or closed reduction. But, — there was a fly in the ointment, — the owner's signed authorization was needed before any surgery could be done, — and no one had come forward to claim the cat. The cat was hospitalized and medicated over the next few days while the staff searched for the owner. They canvassed the neighborhood, put up posters, and placed notices in the local newspaper, — all was done to no avail. It was beginning to look like the little guy was purposely dropped off and abandoned by someone. Four days quickly passed and still no owner, the surgery needed to be performed, and a decision had to be made. I couldn't wait any longer, so I decided to take full responsibility for the cat and do the required surgery. The little guy needed a real name though, instead of just being referred to as, — "the cat". I'd been calling him, "Crash". — It seemed very fitting, because that's what he'd been through. Everybody agreed, — so "CRASH" became his official name.

Crash was scheduled for surgery the next day, and I'd elected to perform a closed reduction intramedullary pinning of the fractured pelvis. The procedure entailed making a small skin incision along the brim of the pelvis, then passing a stainless steel rod/pin down through the medullary (marrow) cavity of the bone, aligning the fractured pieces by "feel", and finally seating (screwing) the pin into the harder cortical layer of the bone. Knowing the anatomy and mentally visualizing the procedure as it's taking place is critical for success, — and a little luck doesn't hurt either. I felt good about the surgery, and the post-surgical x-rays confirmed that the pin was perfectly placed, and that the fractured portions of the pelvis were in excellent alignment. Crash's road-rash injuries were then treated, antibiotics given, and he was done.

Crash was an an ideal patient and he healed rapidly, — as most young patients do. He was happy and playful, in spite of having a stainless steel rod holding his pelvis together, and it wasn't a surprise that he'd become a favorite of clients and staff. At eight weeks post-op, x-rays were taken and showed that the fracture had completely healed, and it was now time to remove the rod and find Crash a permanent home. It didn't take very long before that charismatic little guy found a loving family, and he accompanied them to sunny California. All in all, Crash's remarkable recovery was a testament to his incredible will to survive. He was a true "Road Warrior", in every sense of the word, and was an inspiration to all who met him and heard his story. I'm truly thankful that a concerned stranger stopped by the clinic that day and told us about him laying on the road. Her actions helped save Crash's life, and he remains one of my most rewarding cases.

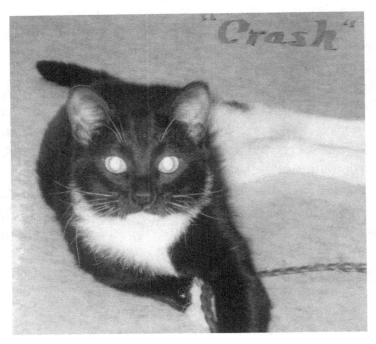

"Crash" the road warrior

Titanium Flash

Perhaps one of the most imposing villains of the cinema was "Jaws" in the James Bond movie, "The Spy Who Loved Me". Jaws had a menacing set of titanium teeth, and he sure knew how to use those things. He definitely was one individual that you wouldn't want to meet in a dark alley. On the other hand, titanium teeth aren't so bad when used for a good reason, and such was the case with an endearing black Labrador Retriever named, "Caly".

Jerod Phillips was an avid outdoorsman who thoroughly enjoyed his hunting and fishing. He loved his dogs too, especially Labrador Retrievers, and spent many hours patiently training them for retrieving downed water fowl. Caly was one of his favorites, and she basically lived to hunt and be with Jerod. She wasn't an overly big Lab either, actually more medium sized, but she was a real dynamo when it came to getting those birds. Jerod, along with his sidekick Caly, occasionally dropped by the clinic for an impromptu visit, just to say, "Hello". Caly knew exactly where the "Cookie drawer" was located, and it didn't matter to her if I was in the exam room with a patient or not, she figured that she was a good girl, deserved some treats, and was determined to stand in front of that drawer and wait patiently until I opened it and delivered the goods. It was rewarding to see clients and patients feel comfortable and enjoy coming to a vet clinic for a change. That was one of my goals. I must admit though, — at times, I tended to "spoil" my patients, — just a tad, — but hey, it was fun! — I had a genuine fondness for my patients.

Jerod stopped by the clinic one day and told me that Caly had recently been showing some reluctance to grab onto (mouth) the downed ducks, and he also noticed that she was refusing to pick up her practice dummy. Jerod went on to say, "Caly has been eating and drinking slower, and that's just not her. She acts like somethin's hurtin'." I told Jerod that I needed to examine Caly, because all kinds of things like dental issues, sores, abscesses, tumors, foreign bodies, nerve problems, and even fractures could account for her acting the way she was acting. We needed to find out specifically what was going on in her mouth.

Caly arrived at the clinic, happy and energetic as usual, acting as if nothing was wrong, — except she didn't go to the treat drawer. I began to examine her mouth, — there were no sores, no abscesses, foreign bodies or tumors, and her teeth appeared to be in relatively good condition, but Caly flinched and pulled her head back when I put pressure on her upper canine teeth. "Ah Hah!" I said to Jerod. "I think I've found her problem. Caly could very likely have an abscessed tooth, and that abscess is causing inflammation and swelling, which in turn is putting pressure on the nerve and surrounding bone. That's what's causing her pain, and that's why she won't hold onto the practice dummy or the ducks. — It's hurts! — It's too painful for her." Jerod asked, "What do we have to do, Doc? She wants to hunt and retrieve, but she can't do it this way. Do we need to pull her teeth? — I'd sure hate to do that, because then she sure as heck couldn't hunt." I told Jerod that root canals would most likely be the only option available for saving Caly's abscessed teeth, but they were pretty pricey procedures. "Doc", Jerod said, Nothin's too pricey for my Caly. I don't care what it costs! If she needs it, — I'll do it for her. When can you do it, Doc?" I told him I didn't have the instruments and equipment necessary to perform root canals, but could refer him to a veterinary dental specialist located in Seattle, some 350 miles away. In the blink of an eye, Jerod said, "Great!" Set me up an appointment." I promptly did just that.

Three weeks had passed, then Jerod called and scheduled a recheck for Caly, as per the dental specialist's recommendations. Caly came bounding into the clinic, her usual happy self, looking for treats — this time. Jerod quickly grabbed Caly, flipped up her gums, and proudly said, "Take a look at those babies, Doc! She's got-em on the uppers and lowers, — they're titanium, — titanium caps, — pretty weird lookin, huh, but she sure feels a lot better — and now she's grabbing stuff again, — no problems, — no pain, — thanks Doc." Caly's shiny new caps instantly reminded me of "Jaws", the huge villain in that James Bond movie, but Caly was no villain, just a real happy camper. The dental specialist had performed root canals on the two upper, (maxillary) canine teeth, then capped them as well as the lower (mandibular) canine teeth. Caly looked tough, but as we all know, — looks can be deceiving.

Caly was an outstanding hunting dog for many years, but when Jerod unfortunately succumbed to a very untimely and tragic accident, Caly suddenly lost her soul-mate and hunting companion. That bond between those two had been broken, and her will to hunt was never the same. Caly lived a few more months, — but then she left to be with Jerod. Sometimes, in my mind's eye, I can see the two of them together again — out there somewhere, — enjoying each others company, — and Caly's titanium teeth flashing in the sun.

Harry Houdini

S omething just wasn't right! Lilly and Mikey, our clinic cats, weren't acting quite themselves. They appeared more apprehensive and hesitated before going upstairs to their main living quarters in the clinic. What also seemed strange was their increased appetites. Their food dish was polished clean, and they usually didn't do that. Something mysterious was going on.

As our business manager, Sandy, was going upstairs to check some archived records, she caught a glimpse of two eyes peering out from under the steps of the stairwell. She was startled momentarily, but then cautiously bent down to take a closer look. The mature face of a grey tabby cat with light green eyes serenely looked back. Sandy asked the cat, "Who are you, and how'd you get in here?". It responded with a soft muffled meow, and slowly emerged from its secure refuge and moved toward her, as if seeking reassurance. The cat was a potent male, about a year and a half old, and actually quite tame. Based on his demeanor, he must have belonged to someone, but why and how did he get into the clinic? That was the big question. Until we had some answers, the cat stayed at the clinic in a comfortable cage, — that was escape-proof.

The search was on to find any possible point of entry. He sure as heck didn't walk through the front door, and there was no way that he could have gotten in through the ventilation system. We kept looking, and eventually found a small triangle shaped opening about 4"x3"x3" in an upper corner of the outside exercise enclosure that we'd built for the clinic cats. At first glance that opening seemed awfully small for a ten pounder to squeeze through, — it would take some determined effort or a little bit of magic to accomplish that feat, — but this cat did it! Some of his grey hair got caught on the fencing and that was the evidence we were looking for. I guess the old saying is true, "Where there's a will, there's a way". Once he'd made it into the exercise enclosure, it was no big deal for him to enter the clinic through the cat door. You'd think that a cat wouldn't want to break INTO a veterinary clinic, but this guy magically found a way inside. So we named him "Harry", — as in Harry Houdini, the renowned escape artist, but our Harry was a reverse Houdini. — He escaped IN!

Before we could find Harry Houdini a permanent home, we needed to test him for Feline AIDS and Feline Leukemia. He was negative to both of those devastating diseases, and that was a huge relief to all of us. The next steps in Harry's "magical makeover" included a bath, getting neutered, vaccinated, dewormed, and microchipped. Harry was now a very handsome cat with a new identity. — It wasn't a surprise to any of us that Harry Houdini soon found a good home,– but it took a bit of magic to accomplish that trick.

"Harry" Houdini

Yellow Jackets

S ummer is a great time of the year, because there are so many fun and exciting things to do. Going to the lake has always been a popular activity enjoyed by people and their dogs. The dogs get to go swimming, fetch things thrown in the water, and even go for boat rides. Everyone's having fun, — until something goes wrong.

There were five lakes within a six mile radius of the veterinary clinic, and I saw my share of summertime emergencies. Everything from fishing hooks and lures embedded in lips and mouths to swallowed triple hooks, cut foot pads, blunt force traumas, eating too much of a good thing, and insect bite reactions. The worst kind of insect bite/sting came from the very aggressive Yellow Jacket wasp. The after effects of such a sting often produced severe reactions, and some of those reactions were even life threatening. There were two dramatic cases which I shall never forget.

A family had come to one of the nearby lakes to do some fishing, and they brought along their two year old buff-colored Cocker Spaniel named, "Trudy". She loved to go out in the boat with the rest of the family. The boat was stocked with all kinds of goodies and refreshments for a day on the water, including a variety of soft drinks, cookies and sliced watermelon. Unfortunately, all those things were sweet, — and they attracted the yellow jacket wasps like crazy. It didn't take long before the pesky yellow jackets were homing in on the boat and the cache of goodies. Trudy did what most dogs would do, – she got annoyed at the marauding insects, and bit at them repeatedly. Suddenly she yelped, — and instantly collapsed in the boat, — unconscious! The family was horror-stricken, and knew that Trudy was in serious trouble, so they quickly raced to shore, got directions to the nearest veterinarian, which was me, and sped into town.

The door of the clinic swung wide open, and a man dressed in shorts and a blue tank top, charged in with a lifeless cocker spaniel dangling in his arms. He frantically hollered, "My dog's been stung by a yellow jacket, — and she's not breathing! I dropped what I was presently doing and immediately went to help the dog. Trudy was in a state of anaphylaxis,(an acute allergic reaction to an antigen -from the sting), she was unconscious, not breathing, and the membranes in her mouth were turning blue from lack of oxygen. She was on the verge of dying! I quickly applied a tourniquet to her left front leg, and attempted to raise a vein, — a very difficult thing to do when the blood pressure is extremely low, — as her's was. The vein didn't raise much, — barely enough for me to see it. I quickly injected dexamethasone and epinephrine intravenously, medications used to counter-act the vascular collapse associated with severe allergic reactions and shock. The distraught family was standing there with me in the room, and as I gave the injections, I told them, "Say a prayer and cross your fingers that this works. I hope we got to her in time". It was really touch-and-go! — It didn't take but a few seconds, and her gums (the membranes in her mouth) started to turn pink again. Trudy then took a breath, and began showing more signs of life. As her respirations continued to increase and she started moving her legs and blinking her eyes, her owners began shedding tears of joy, — and relief. They kept telling me, Thank you, — Thank you, — Thank you".

I hospitalized Trudy for several hours, monitored her recovery, and once she was acting like a normal dog again, I sent her home. I told her family that when Trudy bit at the yellow jacket, it stung her directly into a vein located under the tongue. Trudy had essentially been MAINLINED with the venom of the yellow jacket, and it could have killed her. I also cautioned her owners about the habits of yellow jackets, what attracts them, and what to avoid. Trudy was a very lucky girl to have survived such an ordeal, and hopefully she wouldn't snap at yellow jackets anymore.

Another yellow jacket stinging incident occurred with a seven year old female Bassett Hound named, "Bailey". According to her owner, Janet Artson, Bailey was busily eating her hard food when suddenly she yelped, pulled away from her bowl, and shook her head. Then she started becoming a little wobbly and had, what Janet described as, "a small seizure". Janet went on to say that Bailey's ear quickly swelled up like a balloon, especially the bottom half, and it didn't take long before the skin started looking discolored. This really concerned Janet, so she wanted to have Bailey "checked out" ASAP.

When Bailey arrived at the clinic, it was easy to see why she got stung in the ear. Her long pendulous ears were most likely hanging in and around her food bowl while she was eating, and the yellow jacket wasps were trying to get in on the action at the same time. Both wanted the food, and neither wanted to share. The aggressive wasps must have been aggravated by the floppy ears getting in their way, so they instinctively stung whatever moved, — and it just so happened to be Bailey's ungainly ears. The bottom half of Bailey's left ear didn't look good at all. It was swollen, discolored, and painful to her. There was also a distinct line of demarkation between the healthy and damaged portion of her ear. The wasp venom had caused such a severe allergic reaction within the ear tissue that it eventually resulted in irreparable tissue death. The bottom half of Bailey's ear had to be amputated, —— there was no other feasible option.

Bailey was prepped for surgery, the amputation was successfully completed, and she made a smooth recovery. She was a very good patient with a high pain threshold, and following the surgery, she acted like she hadn't missed a beat. Her head looked a little lopsided though, especially with the bottom half of her left ear missing, but she didn't seem to care. There was, however, one benefit from this incident, — In the future, Bailey only had to be concerned about one ear dangling into her food bowl instead of two.

Not a BB!

A lady and her Australian Cattle Dog, "Tilly", had recently moved from Texas to the Pacific Northwest. The lady had a soft southern accent, and was very knowledgeable about her dog and that particular breed. She'd noticed a small lump with a tiny opening on the dog's side, and assumed that Tilly had somehow been shot with a BB gun. Her concern was that the site might become infected, and she wanted it treated before that happened. Tilly was a very enjoyable patient. She was well behaved, friendly, and nicely groomed. There was definitely an emotional connection between that lady and her dog. Her gentle reassuring touches to Tilly, and the way Tilly gazed back at the lady, it was obvious that love went both ways between those two. I think that's the way the good Lord intended it to be.

I trimmed some of Tilly's hair so that I could get a closer look at the problem area. There it was, — a quarter-sized, raised swelling of the skin with a perfectly round, tiny hole, approximately 3mm in diameter, located smack dab in the center of the lesion. Most of the dogs that I'd seen who'd been recently shot with a BB or pellet gun, showed smaller points of entry, and there usually wasn't that much swelling involved. In this instance, the raised swelling with a small spherical central opening suggested one very likely culprit, — a bot fly or blow fly larvae. Bot fly cases are usually seen in warmer regions of the country, and cause skin problems in cows, horses, and occasionally in people. I'd seen several cows with embedded Bot fly larvae, often referred to as warbles, but I'd never witnessed a dog with that condition. The swelling with the small hole on Tilly's side sure looked like a bot fly case. There was one sure way to find out, — and confirm my diagnosis, — make it wiggle. I deposited several drops of hydrogen peroxide directly into the hole opening, which was the larvae/grub's air hole. The hydrogen peroxide instantly started to foam and bubble up, and it also irritated the embedded larvae, causing it to wiggle and writhe under the skin. The owner and several staff members just couldn't resist taking a closer look at the "larval dance", — and the comments ranged from, "Oh gross!" to "Oh Wow", to "How interesting". It really did look a little sick and weird. There was absolutely no doubt about it. — It wasn't a — BB. — It was a Bot/Blow fly larvae (grub), and that guy needed to be removed, — PRONTO! Embedded grubs or larvae of the bot fly must be carefully removed from the skin. If the larvae were torn or ruptured during the extraction process, toxins from the grub/larvae could potentially be released and enter the patient's bloodstream. That could result in severe allergic reactions and even anaphylactic shock, a serious life-threatening condition.

I administered a sedative to Tilly and used a local anesthetic around the swelling, then proceeded to surgically excise the entire swelling containing the grub. The larvae was removed,— completely and undamaged. It was 3/4 inch long and 3/8 inch wide, — pretty ugly looking too. The owner asked, "How could this have happened?" I told her that a puncture, bruise, or any trauma that compromised the skin tissue could create the ideal place for a bot fly to lay its eggs. When the eggs hatch, the larvae feed on the damaged tissue, and the larvae grow. In time the larvae emerges, drops to the ground, and a young bot fly comes out. Tilly most likely had some sort of initial injury that set the whole scenario into motion.

Tilly was my first, and last dog-bot fly larvae case. I kept the grub/larvae in a small formalin filled specimen jar, and frequently used it as a teaching aid for both clients and students. Believe me, — it was effective!

Song Relief

It's been said that certain strains of music can calm the restless spirits and soothe the troubled minds of humans as well as animals. I'd found that to be true, not only for myself, but for a couple of my patients too.

The Alverez family loved their two Bassett Hounds, and those lucky dogs lacked for nothing. Their names were Heckel and Jeckel, and in all honesty, they were quite spoiled, but nice dogs nonetheless. There was one big problem though, and that was their incessant baying when they visited the clinic. They were happy and excited, — but unfortunately let everyone within a half mile, know it too. Their baying was loud, distracting, ear piercing, and unsettling to all the other animals on the premises. To any pedestrian outside the clinic, it must have sounded like a full fledged fox hunt going on inside, with Heckle and Jeckel in hot pursuit of their quarry.

The odd thing about the whole baying issue was the tonal pitch of the howl. It may sound weird, but the sound frequency of their baying made my ears itch. There I was, attempting to examine these two happy, excitable Bassett Hounds, and all the while they were loudly howling next to my head. My ears started itching like crazy, and in order to maintain my sanity, — I started singing and humming, — anything! Heck, if I didn't know the words, I just made up new ones, kind of, — musical improvisation. An amazing thing happened when I started singing, — the baying stopped, and my ears miraculously stopped itching too. I'd sing stuff like,

"Over the river and through the the woods, — Heckel and Jeckel did go, — they went to the lit–tle vet-nary clinic through ice and drifted snoooo—oh". The dogs looked at me like I'd just lost my mind. — I was getting pretty close to doing just that, — but it worked! — They were quiet, or at least quieter, — and I was able to continue the exams without having my ears assaulted. Over the next several years, whenever Heckel and Jeckkel visited the clinic, I had to sing to them in order to keep the decibels at a manageable level, — and it worked every time! My ears didn't itch, and the Alverez family appreciated the noise relief too.

The day had come when the Alverez family, along with Heckel and Jeckel, were being relocated to the Seattle area. Mr. Alverez had gotten a job promotion, and although they liked the Medical Lake area, the opportunity was too good to pass up. Mrs. Alverez was concerned about how the move would affect their dogs, so she came to the clinic and solemnly inquired, "Do you know of, or could you recommend any singing veterinarians in the Seattle area?" I smiled and said, "No. — I think I'm the only one who sings to his patients". Mrs. Alverez responded, "Oh, I wish there was one, —because they were so good for you when you sang to them". I nodded my head in agreement, and thought to myself, "Sometimes you gotta do what works".

Built on Friday

Sometimes a car that turns out to be a real "lemon", is referred to as a car that was built on Friday. — Meaning that those responsible for assembling the car were more concerned about the weekend than building a car. That "Friday Focus Lapse" often resulted in a car that was haphazardly put together, — and had problems. Unfortunately, assembly foibles can also occur with humans and animals.

The owner, with tears in her eyes, gently and lovingly placed the kitten on the exam table and asked, "Should I have her put to sleep? Is it cruel for me to keep her alive?" I told the lady that I'd check the kitten over first, then give her my honest opinion. There before me was a cute little white kitten, about eight weeks old, and it was plain to see that she had some major physical birth defects. "Snowflake" was the kitten's name, and she moved around on the exam table in a manner suggesting complete unawareness of any physical challenges. She had a totally white hair coat, and big blue eyes, — a genetic combination that is often associated with deafness in cats. When I tested Snowflakes's hearing by having a veterinary assistant blow on a whistle,— Snowflake didn't re-spond, and it was glaringly obvious that her hearing was impaired. Her meow was also rather loud and harsh, — another finding with deaf cats. Not only was little Snowflake hard of hearing, but she also had a severely deformed right front leg that was abnormally short, withered, and shaped in the form of a hook. There wasn't much of a paw either, just a small rudimentary foot pad with only two small nubs masquerading as toes. Her left front leg was much shorter than normal too, but not as drastically deformed as the right front leg. Snowflake was able to stand and support her weight on her left front leg, but not her right. On top of all that, her hind legs were longer than normal, and together with the short front legs, Snowflake looked as if she was perpetually hopping downhill. She didn't seem to mind though, — to her, that was "the normal". Snowflake simply had that unflappable, — "No big deal" attitude.

I told the owner that Snowflake had some genetic and con-genital defects, and although she looked like she was "built on a Friday", she had nonetheless adjusted and adapted extremely well to her physical challenges. Snowflake didn't walk like a "normal" cat either. Instead, she hopped like a rabbit, and played with her toys by hooking and grasping them with her deformed right front leg. She was enjoying life, and I told her owner that in my opin-ion, Snowflake wasn't suffering at all, and she should be allowed to live out her life, — her way.

Snowflake had adapted amazingly well to her physical dis-abilities/challenges, and did in fact live a good life. That happy-go-lucky, affectionate cat, with a "can-do" attitude was a true inspiration, not only to us, but to everyone who had the pleasure of seeing and meeting her.

On the Road Again

Mary Chorde was driving down the I-90 freeway with only ten miles to go before arriving at home. It had been a long day for Mary, and the last thing she expected to see that summer afternoon was a scared little dog running alongside the road. But there it was, and Mary came to its rescue,— because of her genuine passion for dogs. She quickly pulled to the side of the road, put on the emergency flashers, got out of the car, and started calling out to the scampering little canine. It took a little doing, but Mary eventually managed to befriend the frightened dog, and finally held the trembling little guy in her reassuring arms. The little dog was obviously lost, and Mary, knowing that she couldn't just leave the dog alone, way out there in nowhere, decided to take the little guy home with her, and try to find its owner later on.

A week had passed, and in spite of Mary's most ardent efforts, no owner was found. It was beginning to look as if the little dog had found a new home, — with Mary, so she brought her new acquisition to the veterinary clinic for a check-up and vaccinations. I asked Mary if the dog had a name, and she told me that she'd decided to name the dog, "Freeway", because that's where she'd found him. He was a fairly young, bright-eyed, lean and energetic little dog that looked a lot like a purebred Silky Terrier. He also appeared to be well groomed and in good physical health overall. The big question was, "How did a purebred Silky Terrier get so lost, and end up running alongside the interstate highway miles from any city or town?" It just so happened that there was a freeway rest stop about two miles from the location where Mary found him. His previous owners had most likely stopped at the rest stop, and let Freeway stretch his legs, —— and stretch'em he did! — He ran, — and Silky Terriers like to run, — anywhere! He was a defiant, very independent little cuss, and when his owners let him take a little run, well, he kept running, — and running, — and running! I'm sure they looked for him, but he was long gone. They must have been heartbroken. As time waned and their dog couldn't be found, his owners reluctantly had to leave him behind. Freeway was now on his own and had to fend for himself. Fortunately, Mary came along and her love for animals essentially saved his life.

Mary lived two blocks down the street from my house, and I'll never forget the day when a little grey, black and tan colored dog came streaking down the street, — his head up high with fine hair flying in the breeze, and legs moving so fast that they were simply a blur. As he was running past my driveway I yelled out, "FREEWAY"! He stopped dead in his tracks, — and looked straight at me. I pointed in the direction of his house and sternly commanded, "YOU – GO – HOME". He turned his head, — looked towards his home, — then looked at me again, — then took off running in the OPPOSITE direction. The line from the movie, Alice In Wonderland, ran though my head, "I'm late, I'm late. for a very important date. No time to say, hello – goodbye, I'm late, I'm late, I'm late". That was Freeway's modus operandi, and that's probably how he got lost in the first place.

Freeway eventually found his way home, thank goodness. I'll always remember him as a friendly little dog who was very strong-willed. A dog who loved to run, — AWAY, — on the road, ———— again!

"Freeway", the runner!

A Tale of a Tail

The location of a cat's battle scars reveal whether it's a lover or a fighter. Fighters usually have wounds around the head and neck as a result of head-on confrontations, while lovers invariably have "get-away" wounds on the hind end and tail. Miss Priss, a four year old silver tipped Persian cat, was, as her name implied, definitely NOT a fighter.

I first met Miss Priss for a second opinion involving an ongoing, chronic tail condition. Her owners, Al and Beth Dohr, told me that the problem started about two months earlier when the little lady stealthily slipped outside one day to, "see what the real world was like". She found out very quickly that there are some very mean and scary street cats out there. Miss Priss didn't want any part of that action because she was a pampered girl, not a fighter. As she took off running for the safety of home, the neighborhood "bully" cat swatted her on the caboose, and his sharp claws sunk deep into her tail.

The Dohrs were understandably relieved when Miss Priss finally returned home. She appeared frightened, a bit disheveled, and there were a few drops of blood near the base of her tail. Over the next several days, Miss Priss' appetite tapered off, she became less active, and seemed to sleep a lot more. That concerned Al and Beth, so they took her to their regular veterinarian to be checked over. They were told by the vet that Miss Priss had an elevated temperature of 103 F, her tail was infected, and she needed to be placed on antibiotics. The infection, however, did not respond to the antibiotic therapy, and within days a full blown abscess developed. The veterinarian treated the abscess, but the tissue damage was very extensive, and the eventual outcome didn't look very promising. In time, the veterinarian elected to amputate Miss Priss' tail. The amputation site healed well, but Miss Priss licked the tail stump incessantly. There were times, according to her owners, when she'd be quietly sitting on a living room chair, then suddenly go at her tail, — vigorously licking and chewing at it. Al and Beth knew something wasn't right, so they took Miss Priss back to their veterinarian and were told that she was merely adjusting to the tail being gone, and eventually she'd get better and stop licking, — but she never did. That's when the Dohrs sought a second opinion, and brought Miss Priss to me,

The Dohrs entered the exam room and placed a petite and shy little persian cat on the exam table. As they were explaining Miss Priss' history and present condition, I simply observed the cat's mannerism and behavior. She was a gentle little girl, and laid quietly where she was placed. Suddenly, as if "shocked", she swung around and started frantically licking and chewing at her tail stump. Mrs. Dohr sternly said, "Miss Priss,— stop that". I took a closer look at the tail stump and noticed that there wasn't much of a tissue cushion between the remaining tail vertebrae and the skin. I told the owners that Miss Priss could be experiencing discomfort at the amputation site because of adhesions or a neuritis (nerve inflammation), causing a hyperesthesia (excessive sensitivity), and that would explain her sudden and spontaneous reactions, — as if being shocked. I recommended that the tail be amputated at the next vertebrae, and a tissue cushion be reconstructed over the end of the remaining bone. Miss Priss would definitely look like a Manx cat then, — because she'd end up with almost no tail at all. I told Mr. and Mrs. Dohr that the surgery could likely solve the problem. Mr. Dohr asked me, "When can you do the surgery, Doc? She's miserable most of the time, and we hate to see her go on this way." The surgery was quickly scheduled for the next morning.

Miss Priss was the first surgery of the day. She was placed under a general anesthetic, the surgical site was shaved and prepped, and the procedure began. The end vertebrae was removed, and I reconstructed a nice tissue cushion over the remaining vertebrae. She now had a protective layer between the bone and the skin, and hopefully she'd be more comfortable.

Miss Priss made an uneventful recovery, healed quickly, and never licked or chewed at her tail, — or what was left back there,— ever again. Miss Priss once had a beautiful, long, fluffy tail, but now she was much more comfortable with her new look, — and so were Mr. and Mrs. Dohr.

An Overcomer

All if us, mankind as well as animals, often face life alter-
ing health issues. We have a choice of how we respond to
those challenges, — either give in to the problem, or rise up and
triumph over adversity. Sandy, an eight year old, buff-colored
Cocker Spaniel, was an inspiring example of courage and determination. She was a true overcomer.

Judy Granger had noticed that Sandy's eyes were looking a bit
bloodshot that hot, dry summer, and also observed that Sandy was
rubbing her eyes with her paws and on the carpet a lot more than
usual. Judy understandably assumed that allergies were causing
Sandy's eyes to itch, and rubbing them was just a natural response
to the irritation. Judy frequently washed Sandy's face with a damp
washcloth and often scolded her to, "stop rubbing", hoping the
problem would go away, — but it never did. In fact, the eye rubbing seemed to be getting worse, and had become an obsession.
That's when Judy brought Sandy to the clinic for some help.

Sandy was a good patient. She sat quietly on the exam table,
knowing that she'd get treats if she was a good girl, — she was, —
and she did. As I began to examine Sandy's eyes, I noticed that her
right eye was more involved than the left. The sclera (white portion) was reddened, and the eyeball itself appeared swollen and
enlarged. The cornea looked slightly cloudy and steamy because
of the edema that had resulted from the constant irritation of rubbing. The lens, however, was clear, so she didn't appear to have
cataracts. I told Mrs. Granger that Sandy's problems didn't appear

to be an allergy issue, and I needed to conduct several more tests in order to help clarify some of my concerns. I applied a topical anesthetic to her right eye, then used a chartreuse colored stain to check for any corneal ulcers or abrasions. None were found. Next I used an instrument to check the intraocular(within the eyeball) pressure, because the eyeball appeared to be bulging. The pressure was definitely elevated, — not good news. Sandy had glaucoma, an eye condition where there is increased fluid pressure within the eyeball, and it could gradually lead to blindness, or even worse, result in the loss of the eye itself. Mrs. Granger understood the gravity of the diagnosis, and asked if anything could be done for Sandy. I told her that Sandy needed to be placed on some medication to help regulate the intraocular pressure, but sometimes, if the condition had become too advanced, then the medication wouldn't have any effect. If that were to happen, then the intraocular pressure would continue to build, there'd be much more discomfort, and it would then be necessary to remove the eye. Mrs. Granger was willing to try the medication, and accepted the fact that Sandy could lose her eye.

Mrs. Granger faithfully gave Sandy her medication for several weeks, but there was no improvement. The eye, in fact, had actually become larger, and much more painful for Sandy. Her appetite had drastically decreased, she'd become less active and sought seclusion. It was quite apparent that she could not go on this way. The eye had progressed to the point where it couldn't be saved. The decision was made to remove the eye as soon as possible, and the enucleation surgery was quickly scheduled for the very next day. Sandy was the first surgical case that morning. She was placed under a general anesthetic, the surgical site was shaved and prepped, and the painful blind eye was successfully removed. When Sandy awoke from the anesthetic, she acted relieved that the painful eye was gone. Sandy made a speedy recovery, and after all her hair had grown back, it was hard to tell that she only had one eye. There was no rubbing, she was happy, more active and playful, — even played fetch with the ball, her appetite was back to normal, and she was essentially back to her old self, — minus an eye. Everyone was pleased at how well she had adapted.

Several months had passed, and then the remaining eye started to swell. It become reddened, and seemed painful to Sandy. My chief concern had become a reality. The remaining eye had also developed glaucoma, and it too did not respond to medical treatment. With each passing day, Sandy was experiencing more and more discomfort as the intraocular pressure continued to increase. She'd become virtually blind, was in constant agony from the pain, and I was faced with the distinct possibility of removing her only remaining eye. The big question was, "How would she adapt to being totally blind?" Her "Can do" attitude and easy going personality gave me reason to be optimistic about the removal of her remaining eye. I knew that Sandy was an overcomer, and I was confident she'd find a positive way to deal with the absence of eyes, — but it was, nonetheless, a big gamble.

The surgery went well, but now this sweet little dog didn't have any eyes at all. The gradual onset of glaucoma in Sandy's remaining eye had allowed her to adapt to her progressively diminishing eyesight. She'd learned to rely more on her other senses to compensate for lack of vision. She'd turn and tilt her head, listen intently, and elevate her nose to sniff the air for any olfactory clues. If she'd bump into something, — no problem, — she'd back up, reassess, make adjustments, and try again, — totally undaunted. She was still happy and enjoyed life, in spite of the "minor" inconvenience.

You couldn't help but marvel at the courage, true grit, and heart of this little dog with no eyes. Sandy was amazing! She was the perfect example of how an individual can adapt to a setback or physical challenge, and triumphantly overcome. Sandy will always be a special friend and patient to me. — One who really touched my heart and reaffirmed why I chose to become a veterinarian.

"Sandy", the overcomer

A Grand Dame Named Belle

S ome things in life are planned, – some aren't. Accidents can and do happen, – that's for sure. I recall one particularly unfortunate incident where it wasn't an accident, – just poor planning and bad judgment.

"Belle", a 10 year old Labrador Retriever, – about 75 years of age in human years, was considered a senior citizen of the canine world, and the grey hairs on her head and muzzle attested to that fact. Her eyes were slightly dimmed from the pre-cataract condition called bilateral nuclear sclerosis, but that didn't seem to alter her gentle, sweet, and trusting countenance. Although her owners, a young married couple, claimed that she was a purebred Labrador Retriever with "papers", – her light tan hair coat and longish, drooping ears didn't quite fit the typical characteristics of the breed, – but that really didn't seem to matter.

Belle was on the schedule as our 1:20 PM appointment. She walked into the clinic with some difficulty that afternoon, – slowly, – appearing as if she were carrying the weight of the world on her shoulders, – head down, waddling, and seemingly oblivious to her surroundings. At first glance, – she looked as if she'd swallowed a beach ball, – a big one. Not a good sign! We got her on the scales, – 82 pounds, and her temperature topped out at 103 degrees, – definitely elevated. That helped shed some light on why she was acting the way she was. Belle was pregnant, – very pregnant. She'd been used, and was still being used as a breeder by the young couple. They were hoping to get a few more litters out of the ole gal, because they were counting on selling the puppies as a source of additional income. They didn't realize that Belle was past her prime as a viable puppy maker, – way past! "When was she due?" I asked. "Last week." The young man answered. "She looked like she was going to have em' a couple days ago, – she strained a few times, – but then, – nothing. We thought she wasn't ready yet. – Then she stopped eating, – didn't drink much either, – just kind of laid around. We thought something wasn't right and she needed to be checked over."

"Let's see what's going on here, Belle." I said as I began examining the subdued pregnant senior citizen. She had a tired and sad expression on her face, – kind of that, "I give up!" listless and depressed look. The mucous membranes in her mouth were somewhat dry and tacky to the touch, instead of normally being moist and slick, – plus the membranes were off colored instead of being pink. The skin on the back of her neck was slow to return with the "pinch test", – her lungs were clear, but her heart rate was slow. I couldn't detect any sounds or puppy movements in the uterus either, and there was very little swelling of her mammary glands. I laid down the stethoscope, gently patted Belle on the head, – and spoke directly to the young couple. "Belle's in big trouble! – She's dehydrated, – is showing signs of being toxic, – and she may have some dead puppies inside. The long and the short of all this is, – she needs help, – NOW" "What could have caused this, doc?" The young man asked with definite concern in his voice. "Most likely," I answered, "she developed a uterine inertia, – where the uterine muscles sort of, – poop out, and when that happens, the contractions are too weak to expel the puppies. You see, as the time approaches for birthing, – the puppies inside have grown to a point where they aren't getting enough nourishment from mom, and that's stressful to those little guys. The "Red Light" starts blinking, "MAY DAY, – MAY DAY, – we've got a problem Houston!" Their little bodies respond by releasing stress hormones that cross over into the mother's blood stream – and that causes the mother's body to release oxytocin, a chemical which in turn causes the muscles of the uterus to contract, and milk to be let down. End result, – the puppies get the "boot", – and are pushed out. That's the way it's supposed to work, – but sometimes things don't go as planned. One of the big concerns with older dogs getting pregnant is that their hormone levels tend to be lower and less responsive than with younger dogs, and that can lead to some serious birthing problems. – That seems to be the case with Belle. We don't have a lot of time to waste here, – Belle needs a caesarian section, – PRONTO, or else she's not going to make it, and neither will any of the puppies, – if any are still alive in there. – I can't feel any movement, and that's not a good sign. We don't know the condition of the uterus either. Sometimes, in situations like this, the uterus can be severely compromised, damaged, and have areas that aren't even viable, – and in that case, the uterus must be removed in order to save the life of the mother. One thing for sure, – if nothing is done, Belle will surely die" "When can you do this doc?" The young man asked. "Right now!" I told him, "Belle's situation is considered an emergency, – and we've got to get in there right away!." "O.K. doc, – let's do it." They quickly signed the surgical release forms, – and we were off and running.

Belle didn't look good, – and saying that she was a surgical risk was definitely an understatement. First things first though, – IV catheters were placed, the IV line was connected and patent, and within a few seconds, Lactated Ringers fluids were flowing down the line and into Belle's dehydrated body. Next, – she was carefully given a general anesthetic, and quickly entered La-La land, – out like a light, – normal respirations, – everything looked great, – ready to go, – we had to move fast! It didn't take long to get her shaved, prepped, and draped for surgery. All hands were on deck, – three veterinary assistants, and even our receptionist was ready and willing to lend a hand if needed.

The initial skin incision along the ventral midline was a long one. – It had to be that length, in order to provide good exposure and clear access to the grossly swollen uterus. Next, – a delicate incision was made through the stretched Linea Alba, – exposing the abdomen and its contents. The gravid uterus was right there, – and my suspicions were quickly confirmed. This was BAD! – A healthy uterus is normally light pink in color, – but this one had multifocal areas that were dark blue to black, – very unhealthy, – not viable, – unable to be saved. The likelihood of getting a live puppy out of that grossly devitalized uterus wasn't good, – but I proceeded with hopes of saving a puppy or two, however, the thing that took precedence was saving Belle's life. Next, I draped off the uterus with sterile surgical towels, to prevent contamination, and made an incision directly into the body of the uterus, – to gain access to the puppies. "Everybody ready!" I said. "I'll have a puppy for ya in a few seconds." When I grasped the first puppy, – it was limp and unresponsive, – the handwriting was definitely on the wall. As I carefully removed the tiny pup from its quiet sanctuary, it was glaringly obvious that the little guy was beyond help. I gently handed the lifeless body to one of our veterinary assistants, and somberly said, "This ones a goner." Unfortunately, the next pup presented the same scenario. Things weren't looking good, – but I remained optimistic. While maneuvering the next puppy into position, – I felt one of its legs move. "Hey, – I think we've got a live one here! – I need somebody to give this little guy some Dopram (a respiratory stimulant) and start CPR. – Be sure to suction out as much fluid from his mouth as you can." I grasped the puppy, – clamped the cord, and quickly handed him to Carrie, one of our veterinary assistants. She immediately injected 0.2ml of Dopram into the underside of the pup's tongue, –suctioned its mouth, and began giving the little guy CPR. It wasn't but a few seconds before we heard that beautiful squeak/squeal cry coming from a LIVE little puppy. That screechy sound was music to everybody's ears! Yeah-hoos erupted and smiling eyes peering over surgical masks appeared everywhere in that surgery room. The now wiggling, vocalizing little puppy was quickly passed off to the next assistant, who vigorously rubbed, stimulated, and dried off the newborn before placing it into a warming box under a heat lamp.

We repeated that series of procedures five more times, – and managed to deliver five more LIVE puppies. All totaled, – six live puppies, and a mom teetering on the edge. It was nothing short of a miracle, – considering all the negatives in this case. The compromised uterus, with areas of devitalized, necrotic and gangrenous tissue, had to be removed in order to save Belle's life. There was no other option. The compromised uterus was carefully removed surgically, and a four layered closure was used to put Belle back together again. She was also placed on antibiotics, pain meds, and continued to receive I.V. fluids throughout her recovery from the anesthesia. When Belle was fully awake, the noisy little munchkins were placed next to her. She was a very good mom. Although she was still a little on the sleepy side, she instantly began nuzzling and licking the pups. It was really a heartwarming scene to witness.

In the end, – the young owners were pleased that Belle had survived, and that they had six puppies to later sell. However, they were, – to put it mildly, – less than thrilled that the uterus, the "puppy maker", had to be removed. Their "Cash Cow" was no more! The young couple was so upset, in fact, that they refused to pay their bill, and even threatened to sue for loss of potential future income from puppy sales. Oh, bye the way, Belle made a full and complete recovery, was an exceptional mother, and all six puppies thrived and were later sold. Ah yes, – we never saw Belle nor her young owners ever again, and the law suit never materialized. As is often said, "different strokes for different folks". Go figure!

Flatus Maximus

A lunch or dinner composed mainly of beans, lentils, cabbage, or Brussels sprouts can unleash enough intestinal gas to launch a person into orbit. Then there's the associated discomfort from all that pent up methane, which can be pretty intense, —making a bad situation much worse. On a pain scale of 1 to 10, 10 being the most severe, it can often be an 11. Now, – with all that in mind, it's easy to see why an animal experiencing "bloat" (a build up of intestinal gases) desperately needs help and relief, – BIG TIME!

Cows, goats, and sheep, – in fact, all ruminants, burp and belch – a lot! That's a good thing. It's normal, – and necessary. You see, eating all those veggies, like lush green clover and succulent alfalfa, and then the digestive processing of all that stuff, ends up with the production of beaucoup amounts of gas. That gas needs to get out of the rumen, somehow, – and if it can't, then we've got a life threatening situation going on, and it's time to call the vet.

Jeff Childers had a nice little ranch, – about 100 acres or so, just a few miles out of town. It was his "escape" place from his regular day job in the big city. – Kind of a refuge from the pressures of life. It was beautiful, – a rustic styled home nestled amongst the ponderosa pines, a small pond surrounded by cattails nearby, and a meadow of lush green grass and alfalfa in the distance, – very scenic and peaceful. But, – as we all know, trouble can also raise its ugly head, – anywhere, – even in paradise.

There is nothing like walking into the clinic at 7:30 Monday morning, and being greeted by the phone ringing off the hook plus seeing stressed expressions on the staff members' faces. Who needs coffee, – there's already a palpable adrenaline rush permeating the place. One's heart rate immediately steps up a notch or two in anticipation of the ensuing onslaught. "Hey Doc," – get your skates on, – you're really going to need them today." "Great! Whatta we got?" I asked. "Jeff Childers just called, and he's got a cow that's standing out in the pasture, and she looks like a balloon that's ready to pop. She doesn't look good, – according to him. He said that she's huge, and he doesn't think she'll make it, – if she isn't seen right away." An advanced case of bloat is always considered an emergency, – so, I quickly told Donna, our receptionist, "I've got to get out there right now, or else Jeff's gonna have himself a dead cow!" I quickly grabbed my stuff, – told Donna to get on the phone and start rescheduling my appointments, – then jumped in the rig and headed out.

The drive to Jeff's place was kind of a mixed bag, – a beautiful Spring morning, – the sun was shining brightly, – Canadian geese were flying overhead, – but, there was an animal in very serious trouble at the end of the road. I kept the "pedal to the metal", so to speak, because time was of essence for survival. As I pulled up to the home, Jeff was standing on the front deck, – anxiously waiting my arrival. I rolled down the window and asked him, "Where's she at?" "Out in the meadow." He replied. "Hop in, – let's go. Can we catch her?" "She's not movin." He said. As we drove out through that lush pasture, it wasn't hard spotting that cow. There she stood, – head extended, – mouth open, – desperately trying to breathe, – legs spread and belly all ballooned out. She was in major trouble. "You got a trochar Doc? – Should we stick her?" (A trocar is a wicked looking instrument. It is essentially a flanged stainless steel tube, about ½ inch in diameter, and about 6 inches long, containing a huge, removable spike affixed to a handle. The device can be used with "free gas" bloat cases by thrusting it through the skin, into the rumen on the upper left side of the animal, near the pelvis. The spike is withdrawn, leaving the flanged tube in place to release the pent-up gas, and relieve the bloat.). "No!" I said. "Trocars only work with "Free Gas" bloat cases. What we've got here is most likely a case of "Frothy" bloat. "How's that happen, Doc?" "Well" I said. "Eating too much of a good thing, – too much,– too soon. Eating lush, juicy grass, alfalfa, and clover, especially at this time of year, when their G. I. tract hasn't had enough time to properly adjust to all that fresh, succulent green stuff, can end up causing some big problems. They have trouble digesting it, – it gets slimy, – methane gas is given off during the digestive processing of all that stuff and it gets trapped in the slime, – and then you get all that gassy foam and froth building up in the rumen. The cows can't belch off that trapped gas, – so as it continues to build up, – the pressure can become extremely intense, – stretching out the rumen, and making it hard to breathe. It can get really bad sometimes, and if it goes untreated, the animal could even die. What we need to do is get some medicine down into the rumen that breaks up the surface tension of the bubbles, freeing up the gas, and then it can be belched off."

I grabbed a stomach tube, hand pump, mouth speculum, and a bucket, –to which I added about a gallon of water, and a small bottle of bloat treatment medication. Jeff put a rope around the cow's neck so that she couldn't get away, but that wasn't too likely because the poor gal was is such bad shape. I got the mouth speculum in position, and started passing the tube. The cow didn't protest too much, thankfully, and that made the procedure a whole lot easier. I could feel a slight resistance on the tube as it passed down the esophagus on its way to the rumen. "You in Doc?"

"Yeah, –but I haven't reached the rumen yet. When I hit it, a lit-tle gas will come out of the tube, and then I'll have you connect the pump to the tube, and start pumping the stuff into her.—Get ready." We didn't have to wait very long before some raunchy smelling gas came out the end of the tube. "Start pumping Jeff! I said. Jeff's hands were shaking a bit, but he managed to make the connection and started pumping away. "That's it Doc. – I got it all in." When Jeff disconnected the pump, he was rewarded with a good shot of methane gas jettisoning out the end of the tube. "WHEW, – that stuff stinks to high heaven, but I'm glad it's com-ing out of there!" Jeff said while squinting his eyes and pursing his lips. "Don't light a match Jeff", I said. – "Because we'd all go up in flames." He smiled and nodded in agreement. I then pulled out the stomach tube and removed the mouth speculum. "Jeff, – now we've got to get her moving around to help stimulate things, and get that medicine working." Jeff hopped to it, – and with some loud, colorful, words of encouragement together with some tail twisting and a few swats to the rear end, he got the cow to start walking, and it wasn't long before she belched a "good one". "It's workin, Doc!" Jeff said with a tone of relief in his voice. "She's lookin better already." That's what I wanted to hear.

Before heading back to the clinic, I gave Jeff a few words of advice. "Hey Jeff, – here are some things you need to keep in mind to prevent this from happening again. You've got to slowly introduce your cattle to all this lush foliage. That means you can't just put them out there and let them free graze right away. Keep them corralled, give them some dry feed before letting them out in the lush pasture, and don't leave them out there all day. You've also got to get some "bloat-prevention" blocks for the cattle to lick and chew on. That way they'll be taking in some meds that will help decrease the froth from forming. You might also want to keep some bloat treatment drench on hand, just in case, and give it immediately if you suspect one of your cows is bloating." "O.K. Doc, – Thanks for comin'." The drive back to the clinic was nice, – it always is when things work out well. Ah yes, – life is good!

Cows aren't the only ones in the ruminant family who can be victimized by bloat. The first few lines of the ole folk tune, "Bill Grogan's Goat", nailed it. – "Bill Grogan's goat,– was feelin' fine, – ate 3 red shirts, – from off the line, – he moaned and groaned, – in awful pain, – coughed up the shirts, – and flagged the train." Goats eat stuff, – all kinds of stuff, – stuff that doesn't resemble anything that any self-respecting ruminant would normally eat. When that happens, – problems invariably follow.

Sally Abrams called the clinic and nonchalantly told our receptionist, – "One of my goats is bloated up like a balloon. – he's pretty uncomfortable. – Can the doc come out?" Jen hung up the phone, thinking that I was in the back of the clinic, and not realizing that I was standing right behind her, yelled out, "Hey Doc, – we've got a bloating goat for you to take care of." "Jen, – not so loud. "I said. I'm right here. – Where'd you think I was, – out back in the South 40 or somthin?" "Oh, – sorry Doc, – I just wanted to make sure that you heard." "Oh, I heard alright! – Everyone in town heard. Give Sally a call and tell her I'm on my way."

Sally lived just about a mile out of town, so it didn't take long to get to her place. She had a nice set-up, – a herd of about 20 goats, mainly Nubians, and a llama named "Lester" who towered over his little friends. His job was to be the "watchdog" for his little buddies, – to protect them from the coyotes and any other threatening predator. Let me tell ya, – Lester took his job seriously, – real seriously. You had to be careful around that boy! I know, – from a previous experience with him. I was working on another of Sally's goats at the time, while Lester was standing nearby, munching down some alfalfa pellets, and all the while he was giving me the "stink eye". He suddenly stopped eating, turned and sprinted towards me with his head held high and ears folded back. – I instantly knew something bad was about to happen. Lester's pace increased, – and I didn't retreat fast enough. When Lester got within a couple feet of me, he stopped, snorted, and promptly spit in my face! – A direct hit! Slimy, saliva laden alfalfa pellets went everywhere, – even behind my glasses. Sally quickly got him out of there before he could do some serious damage. – It was really quite funny though, – me standing there with my face covered in llama juice and sticky, wet, alfalfa pellets. The lesson learned, – llamas really do spit, – they can definitely hit the mark, – and don't tick off Lester.

I pulled into the driveway, and could see Sally standing out there in a large cross fenced corral with the rotund little goat in hand. She had attempted to separate the bloated little guy from the others, but that was a bust! Goats were milling around everywhere, – jumping on wooden spools and shelters, – chasing, butting, and sparring with each other, – acting crazy, – and seemingly oblivious to what was going on around them – all except "Lester". "Hi Doc. Thanks for coming. – Oops, – let me put Lester away before we get started." While she was doing that, I got my medical stuff together. The penned area was eaten down and bare of any significant vegetation of any sort, and the goats were being fed good quality grass-alfalfa hay, – so – frothy bloat seemed unlikely. The poor little guy was just standing there quietly, – abdomen distended, head stretched forward, legs spread, – looking pretty uncomfortable. "Hey Sally," I said, – "Looks like he swallowed a basketball or something." "He could have." She replied. "You know, – goats try to eat just about anything that comes their way, – and it wouldn't surprise me if he'd try to down a basketball." The little guy's belly was really swollen, especially on the left side where the rumen is positioned. "Sally," – I'm going to tap the rumen to see if I can get any "free" gas to come off, or see if we're dealing with a "frothy" bloat." Sally held the little goat steady while I quickly thrust a 2 inch 18 gauge needle into his distended left side, – up high, near his pelvis. "Pssssssss" – A long sustained flow of methane gas whistled out through the hub of the needle. I withdrew the mini trocar and said to Sally, "Looks like we've got a "free" gas bloat case here. – Most likely a blockage of some sort. – What could this little guy have gotten into?" – Sally had a puzzled expression on her face. "I don't know what he could have eaten, – I keep the pens pretty clean. – Oh, – wait a minute. – We had some strong winds come through here the other day, – and lots of junk was being blown around." "Did you see any stray garbage bags or something like that flying around?" I asked. "Yeah, – I did, – and some got caught in the fence." Sally replied. "I guess he could have chewed on those things, – huh? – What do you think, Doc?" "Well," I said. "The little guy could have eaten some of that stuff, – and it could have gotten hung up in the esophagus, produced an obstruction, and prevented the gases from escaping. I'm going to pass a stomach tube and see if I can dislodge anything that might be causing the blockage, – if there is one. If that's the case, – then we'll get some of the gas to come out of the tube, and that'll decrease the pressure, and make him more comfortable. I'll also drench him with some special meds that will help break up some of the residual gas and get things moving." "Sounds good to me." Sally said, matter of factly.

I grabbed a flexible stomach tube, placed the small mouth speculum in position, – which the little goat wasn't too thrilled about, and started passing the tube down the esophagus on its way to the target. There was commotion all around us. – Some of the other goats thought my portable medical box was a play thing, and unabashedly started jumping on top of it, – essentially playing, "King Of The Mountain". Sally tried, in vain, to shoo them away, – but, – like any undisciplined kids, – they quickly returned,

– stepping on and in the box, – using it as a launching pad for their aerial gymnastic kick maneuvers. Heck, – they tipped over my medicine bottles, and sent many of my instruments and syringes flying in all directions. It was a zoo! Truthfully, – the whole thing resembled a bizarrely comical scene from some Keystone Cops movie. Nonetheless, – while all this was going on, I somehow managed to successfully pass the stomach tube to the right place. The end of the tube was almost to the rumen when I suddenly detected some moderate resistance to the passage. – "Ah ha!" I said to myself. "the obstruction!" A cautious, but more forceful, thrust of the tube was all that was needed, – and, – "BINGO"! – The resistance stopped, and some raunchy smelling gas instantly came belching out the end of the tube. – Whew! I let as much of the pent up methane gas escape as I possibly could, – then infused the anti-bloat medication directly into the rumen. "Sally", I said. "– "I pushed the obstruction, or whatever was causing the blockage, down into the rumen. It should pass. It felt rather soft, and moved pretty easily, so it probably was a plastic bag or some other debris that had blown in with that strong wind the other day, – and this little guy couldn't resist imbibing!"

The little goat now looked a whole lot thinner, – like he'd lost a couple pant sizes, and he seemed to feel much better too. He even started moving around, and jostled with his buddies, who appeared happy to have their friend back to "normal". Before heading back to the clinic, I gave Sally a few aftercare instructions and cleaned up the mess in my medicine box, – thanks to the antics of the other "helpful" goats. In all honesty, goats are pure fun! They thoroughly enjoy life, and always make farm calls very interesting.

The Lump

One thing's for sure, – a veterinarian's life is never boring! No two days are ever the same, and that's good, because it keeps a person on their toes. You need to be mentally prepared for just about anything in a general practice, including stuff that wasn't even mentioned in veterinary school. A perfect example of a very unusual case involved a cat named "Whiskers".

Checking over the appointment book was one of the first things I did when arriving at the veterinary clinic each morning. A quick glance at what was scheduled helped me get ready for the cases I'd see that day. On one particular day, things looked pretty routine, but the two o'clock appointment caught my eye, – a cat named Whiskers with a lump on the belly. Probably an abscess, small umbilical hernia, or a tumor, I thought to myself. – We'll see.

When I walked into the exam room at 2 pm, I was greeted by a young, grey and white colored tabby cat standing nonchalantly on the exam table. The patient record card stated that it was a seven month old, intact male that wasn't current on its vaccinations, and needed to have a lump on it's belly checked. "Hi Whiskers!" I said. "How ya doin today?" He was a friendly little guy, – purring like crazy, and he even head butted my hand as I approached, looking for some lovin. I gave him a brief physical exam before addressing the main concern for him being at the clinic. His eyes were bright and clear, his ears were clean, mouth and teeth looked good, heart and lungs sounded clear and normal, his hair coat was smooth and shiny, there was no evidence of fleas, and his temperature was in the normal Now, to check the "lump" on his abdomen. Whiskers was standing with his right side toward me, and as I passed my hand over his abdomen, – there wasn't just a "lump", – but instead, – there was a HUGE swelling, about three inches wide and seven inches long. It extended from the zyphoid cartilage of the ribcage, all the way back to his groin. Further palpation {examination by touching and feeling} revealed that it was soft, moveable, with firm edges. Whiskers showed no signs of discomfort throughout the exam, in fact, he acted like he was enjoying the whole thing, – purring, – head butting, and he actually started drooling. Whiskers was a great little patient. I looked up at his owners, a young married couple, and emphatically stated, "Whiskers has some major issues going on here. It's definitely not just a "lump", and it's not a tumor or an abscess either. I believe he has a serious birth defect, – a major structural flaw, – like he was "made on Friday", – late Friday. His abdominal muscles and connective tissue never closed together like they were supposed to do, and as a result, all of his intestines and internal organs are lying just underneath his skin, – not good, – in fact, – pretty dangerous. He'd be in some deep kimchi, – some serious trouble, if he ever got cut or punctured in that area. What we need to do is to rebuild him! Whisker's owners just stood there, – silently, with expressions of shock and disbelief on their faces. Finally the wife spoke softly with some trepidation in her voice. – "How much is this going to cost? – We don't have much money. Can we make payments?" "Well", I said. "There's a lot that has to be done, – the surgery alone is going to be quite extensive, delicate, and time consuming. Whiskers will also receive I.V. fluids throughout the surgery, and will need to be placed on antibiotic therapy post-op. He needs his vaccinations, and heck, – we might as well neuter him at that time too. We'll give you an accurate estimate of the charges, but I can definitely tell you, right now, that we're looking at around a thousand dollars, – plus." The young couple quietly discussed what they were faced with and their options, – then the husband somberly commented, "We can't afford it, – just put him to sleep". Those were the words I didn't want to hear. Quite honestly, – my heart sunk. Putting down a happy, essentially healthy animal that had an excellent chance of living, wasn't an option to me. — I couldn't do that! So, – I told the young couple, – "I'll tell you what, – Whiskers is a loving little friend and family member to you. It isn't his fault that this happened, and he deserves a chance to live. So, — here's what I propose for Whiskers and you guys, – I'll do the surgery, neuter and vaccinate him, – then you can pay off the bill as you're able . – Would you be willing to do something like that?" Tears welled up in the young couples' eyes, and they both uttered simultaneously, – "Thank you." Yeah, — doin stuff like that cost me thousands and thousands of dollars over the years, – giving away services, – but I believe, and continue to believe that the Lord meant what He said, when He told us, "Those who do it unto the least of these, you have done it unto Me." I believe that He rewards and blesses the benevolent works of people who help and value His creatures and His creation, – maybe not financially, but in so many other ways. That's good enough for me.

Whiskers was scheduled for surgery the following day. He had to be NPO (no food -empty stomach) prior to surgery, so, – when we walked into the clinic that next morning, we were greeted by a very vocal little guy, – complaining about the poor food service in that place. He was first up for surgery that day, so he didn't have to wait very long before being placed under a general anesthetic. He was then prepped for surgery, – meaning that a swath, six inches wide, was shaved from his armpits to his groin. Next came a surgical soap scrub, followed by an antiseptic rinse, – IV's were placed, – the surgical area was then draped off, and we were good to go.

The initial skin incision was a long one, – real long, – about eight inches long, – right down the middle of his abdomen. I had to be extremely careful with the scalpel, because Whisker's intestines were positioned just underneath the skin, and nicking those babies would spell disaster! Once the skin was reflected back and held in position with tissue forceps, the defect was clearly visible. Heck, there was at least a two inch gap/separation between the abdominal muscles, and that space extended almost the full length of the incision. The peritoneum, (the thin, transparent membrane that lines the abdominal cavity), which acts something like an inner tube of a bike tire, was adhered (stuck onto) to the muscles instead of being connected by fibrous tissue, like it should have been. I had to very delicately separate the tissue -thin peritoneum from the muscles, then reunite it by using an ultra fine (tiny) suture. Once that "inner tube" was rebuilt, the next procedure was the debridement and reconnection of the edges of the abdominal muscles. To accomplish this, I had to carefully scarify (scrape down to the blood bed, using a scalpel blade) the muscles and then reconnect the muscles by using a stronger suture. After that was completed, next came the process of stabilizing the subcutaneous tissue by using a strong, slow absorbing, suture thread, and finally, – the skin was closed, using a continuous interlocking suture pattern. Everything came together nicely. VIOLA'!!! – we were done with the tough part. Whiskers was then neutered, given an antibiotic injection, pain meds, and placed in a nice warm recovery cage. He woke up a few hours later, – acted like nothing had happened, – ate like he'd never seen food before, and went home the next day.

Whiskers was a great patient, and he healed up nicely, – without any problems. I'm thankful that I closed him with strong sutures, because he was a very active boy, -and was running and jumping around like crazy just two days post-op. Sutures of lesser strength may not have held him together, and that would have created some major problems. He looked a little funny for a few weeks, – with that naked tummy and stitches running from stem to stern, – making his underside resemble a weird looking football, – but, – with "tincture of time", the sutures were removed, – all his hair grew back, – and hey, – he finally looked like any other "normal" healthy cat. Whiskers was happy again, and so were his owners.

"Whiskers"

Hold Your Nose

Perhaps one of the least favorite procedures for veterinarians, vet techs, and the animals themselves is manually expressing or draining the anal glands. Nobody likes doing it, or having it done to them, because the treatment requires placing a gloved finger into a very private place, — where the sun doesn't shine, — and then squeezing. Heck, — inserting a rectal thermometer is bad enough, — but a finger!

The good Lord must have had a great sense of humor when He created those little gems. There are two of those guys, one on each side of the anus, hiding just under the skin, surrounded by the sphincter muscles, and positioned at 4 & 8 o'clock to the caboose. These little aromatic packages produce and secrete a very pungent fluid which is released onto the stools (feces) during defecation (pooping). The "personal" odor of the anal gland secretion is sort of a "calling card" that doubles as a territorial marker, — an aromatic nametag, — so to speak. So, when dogs get around other dogs, there's this "meet and greet" ritual where they go around sniffing each other's butts, — introducing themselves. We've all seen it before, and to many people it is a bit embarrassing to watch. This uninhibited canine "social hello" always makes me thankful and relieved, that as human beings, shaking hands and a smile is still the socially accepted form of introduction.

Sometimes, during moments of high anxiety, fear, and during those "fight or flight" episodes, when the "pucker factor" really kicks in, — those anal glands get suddenly squeezed by the

317

sphincter muscles, and — KA-POW-EE! — everybody gets the drift, – instantly! That nauseating, pee-eooh-ee odor quickly permeates the air at warp speed, and assaults one's sense of smell. That offending odor can sometimes be so bad that you'd swear it could strip the paint off the walls, — but hey, that's the way those babies are supposed to work, — that's their job! The real "thrill", however, comes when those little gems have problems, — like getting blocked, abscessed, or rupturing, leaving open wounds. Sometimes, surgically removing the anal glands is the only way to relieve the pain and suffering. One thing is certain, — anal gland issues are always uncomfortable for the animal, — and they definitely let you know all about it.

One of the tell-tale signs of a dog experiencing anal gland problems is the proverbial "bum scoot"! Ah yes, — modesty goes right out the window. They'll be out there in the front yard, — in front of all the gawking neighbors, or in the living room, —in full view of your house guests, — just doing their thing, — the rear end "carpet dance". It doesn't matter to them who's watching, or what it may look like, — if it feels good and helps to relieve the pressure and make things more comfortable, — just do it! Now, where have we heard that before?

Ideally, the anal gland secretion should be liquid in consistency, for ease of passage through a tiny duct. But, — as we all know, things don't always go as planned. When that happens, a quick trip to the veterinarian is needed to make things better.

I was in my office, working on patient records, when Sharon, our receptionist let me know that the next appointment had arrived. "Hey Doc, you've got a new patient to see. It's a dog named "Rocky", and he's having anal gland problems. He's in exam room one, and ready to be seen. Here are his medical records from the previous vet." A quick glance at the dog's records showed repeated visits to the vet for anal gland issues. As the saying goes, "Fore warned is fore armed".

As I entered the exam room, I was greeted by some "happy howling". Rocky was a four year old Beagle-cross who didn't look much like a Beagle, but that distinctive howl of his left no doubt about Beagle genes being in there somewhere. I introduced myself to the owner, and then to the bright-eyed little dog. "Rocky little buddy, how're ya doin? I hear you're havin' some problems with your caboose." Kathy, his owner, chimed in. "Doctor, — Rocky's having problems with his anal glands again. I've been taking him to the vet at lease twice a year to get those things drained. He's O.K. for a few months, but then he starts licking and dragging his hind end across the grass again. Is there something that can help him so he doesn't have to go through this so much?" I paused for a moment and then told her, "Sometimes increasing the fiber in the diet can be helpful. The extra bulk in the stools has helped other dogs with similar anal gland issues, — but nothing is 100% except death and taxes, — if you know what I mean." Kathy understood, and commented, "I'd be willing to do just about any-thing if it'll help." I held Rocky's head in my hands, looked him straight in the eyes, and told him with a smile, "Now, little buddy, it's time for us to become r-e-a-l-l-y close friends. I call it the IRS handshake procedure." Rocky just stood there, happily wagging his tail, and a look of eager anticipation in his eyes.

Now, the most effective method used to drain anal glands is to insert one's gloved finger into the animal's rectum, — isolate the gland between thumb and finger, — and gently, but firmly squeeze, — and strip out the contents from the gland. Anybody watching the procedure invariably had a squinty-eyed expres-sion on their face and often commented, "Oooh, that's gross," or "Oh my, — I'm sure glad that you're doing that instead of me.". Honestly, — I wasn't all that thrilled about doing it either, — but it had to be done. I'd usually try to interject a little humor into the disgusting routine as I inserted my finger into the animal's rectum. I'd nonchalantly sing, in a half-hearted way, "Over the river and through the woods, — into your heinie we go." That bit of levity usually produced more laughs and giggles than groans, — but the patients weren't amused, although they felt much better when we were done.

Rocky was a good little patient, and he survived the ordeal. Kathy followed my recommendation of increasing the fiber content in Rocky's diet, and pardon the pun, — everything turned out good in the end. Rocky was a whole lot happier, and so was Kathy.

A Stinky Proposition

Cattle are, for the most part, gentle, unassuming creatures, content to just do their own thing, live in the moment, and blow off the cares of this world. Sounds good, until something goes wrong, and when that happens, — well, things begin to implode, in more ways than one. I think we can all identify with that.

Steve Bailey was a successful wheat farmer who also had a small herd of Hereford cows. He was a good farmer and a conscientious cattleman to boot. Not much got by Steve. He ran his cattle on open rangeland most of the year, but corralled and provided shelter for them during the colder winter months. Steve always made sure to have plenty of alfalfa hay available for his cows during those tough times, knowing full well that good feed was critical to getting his cows through those cold, stressful months. However, like the ole saying goes, "the road to hell is paved with good intentions" and although Steve tried to do everything right, some of his cows still had a few health issues.

The phone rang, our receptionist answered, and shortly thereafter, hung up the receiver and relayed the message to me, "Steve Bailey needs you to take a look at one of his cows. He says she's slowed down on her eating and has a big lump under her jaw. He'd like you to come out this morning if you have the time." The schedule was pretty light that day, so I told Rachel to call Steve and tell him to get the cow caught up, and I'd be out to his place in about an hour.

I loaded up my rig with the medications and surgical instruments that would be necessary to diagnose and treat this case, and was on the road in short order. It didn't take long to get to Steve's farm, only about ten miles from the clinic. When I pulled into Steve's driveway, there he was, — standing next to the cow, — caught up and quietly waiting in the squeeze chute next to the corral. That was a welcomed sight, and a relief, because it meant that I didn't have to do my cowboy routine with this cow.

As I was getting my stuff out of the truck, I asked Steve, "When did you first notice the lump under her jaw?" "Oh,— about two weeks age." He said. "I gave her a shot of penicillin, — it got better for a few days, — but then it came back again. She was still eating, but that slowed down a couple days ago too. What d'ya thinks goin on doc?" "There could be several things." I said. "But first I've got to check her temp to see if she's got an active infection going on." The cow's rectal temperature was 103 degrees F, — definitely elevated! "Steve", I said, "I think she's got an infection, very likely an abscess, and I'm going to do a needle tap to see if we've got any pus in there." I grabbed a 16 gauge x 1 ½ inch long needle that resembled a pointed mini-pipe, and quickly thrust it deep into the center of the lump. In the blink of an eye, thick, foul smelling, pinkish-green, nasty looking pus oozed out the hub of the needle. "BINGO!" I said. "We've got a doozy of an abscess here. I've got to check the inside of her mouth for the possibility of a bad tooth or the point of entry of some foreign object." I grasped the cow's big, raspy tongue, pulled it to one side, and took a quick, — very quick look. Believe me, she wasn't too keen about having that done! I told Steve that there didn't seem to be any problem inside her mouth, so the next thing to do was to lance open and drain the abscess. I grabbed the scalpel and made a 3 inch incision on the bottom side of the large lump, so as to get ventral drainage. — BONANZA! — The flood gates opened!!!

Out poured about a quart of thick, putrid smelling, pinkish-green pus, that sort of resembled a certain kind of salad dressing, which incidently, I refuse to eat anymore. The whole gross scene could have gagged a maggot! It was really foul! Steve stood there with a grimacing, pained expression on his face, and while holding his nose closed with his fingers, he blurted out, "ZOWIE! —that's a bad one isn't it doc. What could have caused that?" I told him, "Sometimes cheat grass awns in the hay can penetrate the mucous membranes in a cow's mouth, and then they migrate deep into the tissue. Usually bacteria is carried along with the thorny seed and start growing like crazy in all the blood and serum from the inflammation, — and then you get a doozy of an infection, — and that's what we have here." I tried to get as much pus out of there as possible, then thoroughly cleaned the cavernous wound with an antiseptic solution, and finished up by giving the cow a hefty antibiotic injection. My final instructions to Steve were to keep the incision open, clean, and draining for several days.

That stench remained in my nostrals for most of the day, — but it was all worth it, because the cow was now definitely on the mend.

Follow the Bouncing Ball

Growing up on a farm taught me many things, and one of the most valuable lessons I learned was how to be resourceful. That ability to find quick and imaginative ways to overcome difficulties and challenges not only helped me solve many everyday-type problems, but also became an invaluable asset in my veterinary career.

One of my friends and fellow classmates at Eastern Washington University was Alex Treveno. Alex's family immigrated from Cuba to the United States in the late 50's and made Spokane their new home. Alex was a polite, somewhat reserved, very conscientious and intelligent individual, whose ultimate goal was to enter the field of medical research. That decision was somewhat of a disappointment to his father, who was a very successful and highly respected physician and surgeon. Dr. Trevino would have liked his son to follow in his footsteps, but nonetheless, fully supported and encouraged Alex in his vocational aspirations.

Alex was one of the first people to congratulate me when I got accepted into the Washington State University School of Veterinary Medicine. He was almost as excited as I was. I'll never forget the day Alex showed up at class, carrying a cardboard box full of stuff. He walked over to where I was sitting, and plopped the box down on the chair next to me. A clanking sound resonated from the box, so I asked Alex, "What the heck do you have in there, — a bunch of old car parts?" Alex just shook his head and replied, "Here ya go, I don't know if you can use any of these, but here are some old instruments that dad doesn't use anymore. Some are broken, — some are bent, — anyway, — maybe there's something in here that you can use someday. — The price is right though." I thanked Alex profusely, and opened the box like it was an early Christmas present and excitedly peered inside. The box was filled with all kinds of stainless steel instruments, —an assortment of thumb forceps with bent and missing teeth, — a bunch of small towel clamps that were sprung and didn't close properly, — abdominal retractors and vaginal speculums of various sizes, scalpel handles, and a couple large, 10 inch curved tissue forceps with ratchet grips. Those babies had four, half inch long, pointed, interlocking teeth too. They were wicked looking instruments! I told Alex, "You never know, — someday these instruments may come in pretty handy." I really appreciated the gesture, and I kept that box of misfit instruments for many years. One particular instrument that really caught my eye was that 10" long, curved tissue forceps with the pointed teeth. I kept that thing in the second exam room drawer, — just in case.

"Blitz" was a four year old Alsation, also known as a German Shepherd. He was a highly trained security dog at a nearby international airport. His trainer and handler, Jeff Baker, had previously told me how much time and money was invested into Blitz's training, and needless to say, that was one extremely valuable dog in more ways than one. Jeff and Blitz were inseparable. There was mutual respect between those two, and and they made an outstanding team. One of the training aids that Jeff used with Blitz was an orange-colored, hard rubber ball, about 2 ½ inches in diameter, and extremely responsive, — in other words, — it was SUPER bouncy. Blitz absolutely loved playing with that ball, — and that was the key! Playing with that ball was Blitz's reward for satisfactorily performing an assigned task.

During one of their training sessions, Jeff tossed the ball like he'd done a hundred times before, — but this time disaster struck. The ball had bounced high into the air, and when Blitz jumped up with his mouth opened wide to retrieve the ball, the dense, hard rubber ball flew deep into his mouth, and became instantly stuck in his throat, wedged between the hyoid bones directly in front of his larynx, — effectively blocking Blitz's airway. Blitz made several unsuccessful attempts to cough up the ball, and pawed frantically at his muzzle in an attempt to dislodge the thing, but to no avail. Blitz wasn't getting much air, and he soon collapsed from lack of oxygen. Jeff quickly grabbed Blitz, put him into the car, and raced to the clinic. Thank heavens Jeff lived only about one mile from the clinic, because Blitz didn't have much time left on this earth. Jeff charged through the clinic door with a limp dog in his arms, and immediately yelled out, "He's got a ball stuck in his throat and he can't breathe!" We rushed the two of them into the second exam room, — I quickly grabbed a mouth speculum, and opened Blitz's mouth. I could barely see part of the ball, — it was way down there in his throat. I attempted to manually dislodge the ball, but it wouldn't budge. The ball was locked between the hyoid bones directly in front of the trachea, obstructing the air flow. Blitz's tongue was turning blue in color from the lack of oxygen, — I didn't have much time, — I had to dislodge that ball, — NOW, — or Blitz wasn't going to make it! Then, by what might be perceived as divine inspiration, I remembered that strange looking 10 inch long, curved tissue forceps with those wickedly pointed teeth. The same one that Alex Trevenno had given to me many years ago. I often thought that someday that "thing" would come in pretty handy, — and today was that day! I quickly took it from the drawer, — opened Blitz's mouth, and sunk the pointed teeth of that instrument into the hard rubber ball. As I pulled on the ball to dislodge it, I could feel the hyoid bones and laryngeal cartilage give way. Then, with a more forceful tug, the ball suddenly came loose, and at that precise moment I heard perhaps the most beautiful sound in all the world, — Blitz taking a deep breath, — a breath much overdue, — a breath of life. It didn't take long for Blitz's tongue to pink up, and shortly thereafter he blinked and moved his head. That was a close one!

Blitz made an amazing recovery, and didn't suffer any adverse effects from the short period of oxygen deprivation. Oh yeah, I kept that hard rubber ball, with the four permanent puncture marks, because I didn't want Blitz, nor myself to go through that experience again. That unusual instrument may have laid idly in the drawer for many years, — but it did, eventually, prove to be very useful, and actually turned out to be a real life saver.

Shatzi

The attributes of the "ideal surgeon" during the 15th century were, — to possess the eyes of an eagle, the heart of a lion, and the hands of a woman. Those qualities are every bit as relevant today as they were back then, and there were many opportunities for me to see if I had the "right stuff". Perhaps one of my toughest tests involved a courageous little dog named, "Shatzi".

Shatzi was a gentle spirited, three year old Miniature Schnauzer who could charm the socks off anyone who met her. She was perfectly named too, because the German word, schatz, means little darling or sweetheart, — and this little girl certainly fit the bill. She really knew how to work it, and always managed to schmoose her way into accompanying the Bauers in their family car and motor home. Unfortunately, she liked being in and around vehicles a little too much, and that set the stage for what eventually happened.

Emergencies go with the territory in veterinary medicine, so I wasn't particularly caught off guard when I heard our receptionist answer the phone and say, "Yes, — he's here. Come right in." She then hung up the phone, quickly turned to me and said with a tone of urgency in her voice, "We've got a HBC (hit by car) coming in! They live here in town, and will be here in a few minutes." It wasn't long before Mr. Bauer came through the clinic door, clutching a motionless Shatzi wrapped in a blanket. Mrs. Bauer was at his side, stroking Shatzi's head, — trying to console and comfort the little injured dog. The trio was immediately ushered into the surgery room, where Mr. Bauer gently placed his precious bundle upon the stainless steel surgical table. All the while Mrs. Bauer, with tears welled up in her eyes and trembling hands, kept repeating, "Oh Shatzi, — oh Shatzi, — why'd this have to happen?" Mr. Bauer didn't utter a single word. — He just stood there, choking back tears and staring down at the injured little dog wrapped in a blood soaked blanket.

Shatzi was barely clinging to life. She had delayed reflexes, shallow respirations, falling blood pressure and her mucous membranes were very pale in color, due in part to the large amount of blood that she'd lost. Little Shatzi was also in a state of shock. She was in major trouble, and I had to act fast or she'd be gone! As I lifted part of the blanket to gain access to her right front leg for placement of an I.V. (Intravenous) injection, I caught a glimpse of her severe injuries. — It looked bad! I quickly applied a tourniquet to her leg, elevated the cephalic vein, inserted the needle, and immediately injected medications to counter shock. It was touch and go for a few seconds,, but suddenly Shatzi's respirations normalized, her mucous membranes started pinking up, and she became more active, — moving her head around and blinking her eyes. An I.V. catheter was then placed in the cephalic vein of her left front leg, and Shatzi began receiving life-saving fluids and medications to ease the pain. She was now out of immediate danger and her condition had stabilized. Whew! Once over that hurdle, the next step was to assess her injuries. As I gently removed the blanket from around Shatzi's little body, the full extent of her wounds came into view. At that very moment a chorus of comments, ranging from "Oh my!" to "OMG" to "Oh no" rose up from those witnessing the mangled mess. The skin from the top of her back down to her left flank, and from her last rib to her hindquarters was severely traumatized. The skin was torn and shredded with large portions actually missing! The carnage strangely resembled a badly ripped and torn sail of a ship that had been caught in a violent storm at sea. As bad as it was, — that wasn't the worst of it. The lower half of Shatzi's left hind leg was gone, — totally missing, — with only a few flaps of skin dangling over the exposed, splintered end of her left femur bone. Mr. Bauer looked down at Shatzi, and with a sorrowful, quivering voice asked, "Would it be kinder to put her to sleep?" Before I answered, I quickly glanced at Shatzi, and in spite of her extensive injuries, she still had that, "will to live" glint in her eyes, or at least that's what I perceived. "No" I said. "Let's give her a chance. It won't be easy, and there could be all kinds of complications. It's going to take a long time to recover, even if things go well. Her left hind leg will need to be amputated and multiple surgeries will be necessary to get skin and scar tissue to cover the degloved (where the skin is completely torn away from the underlying tissue) areas. Shatzi is young, and she wants to live, — that's half the battle." Mr. Bauer stood there, — quietly processing the options, — then turned to his wife and asked. "What do you think we should do?" Mrs. Bauer's facial expressions softened as she said with a wistful smile. — "Well, she's part of our family, and she's always been there for us. — We need to be there for her too. — Let's do it!" That comment was good enough for me. I reassured the Bauers that I'd do my best to help Shatzi, — then turned to the little dog who was now quite alert, but unsure of all that was happening around her. "Little lady." I said, "Let's get the show on the road, — we've got a lot of work to do."

Once Shatzi was sufficiently stabilized, a general anesthetic was administered and she was soon snoozing comfortably, — free of pain and breathing normally. X-rays were then taken to check for other broken bones and any evidence of internal complications. No additional breaks were found, — thank goodness, — and she looked good on the inside too. That little girl had enough problems already. Shatzi was then whisked off to surgery prep for triage of her injuries. It was a no-brainer that amputation of the left hind leg was number one on the "to do" list. It would be a challenge because I didn't have much viable skin and tissue to work with. First things first, — Shatzi's wounds were carefully cleaned, debrided, disinfected, and medicated prior to surgery. As I looked down at her little ravaged body, I thought to myself, "This is going to be a long, drawn out process." Much of Shatzi's skin on her left upper side and back was missing, — gone, — and what remained didn't look all that great either, — not a good situation. Honestly, getting her back to where she could enjoy life again would be nothing short of a minor miracle, — but I was hopeful. It was then that an old adage by a 16th century English clergyman came to mind, "You can't make a silk purse out of a sow's ear". He was referring to people who were up against a hopeless task. I didn't think that this case was particularly hopeless, but it sure looked bad, and I knew I had to be on my A-game if I expected to make a "silk purse" out of this mess.

The leg amputation went well, considering the massive trauma, and I managed to reconstruct a nice protective muscle pad over the remaining portion of femur bone. Once that was accomplished, my attention then focused on finding enough healthy skin to cover the surgical site. Believe me, — that was tricky, and there were moments when I wondered how I could pull that off, — not much viable skin to work with. More than once I silently prayed, "Lord, help me get this back together". I had to resort to some "creative" reconstruction procedures, meaning using ANY available skin, — even devitalized skin as a temporary bandage, of sorts, to cover the exposed muscle tissue. I was sweating bullets for almost two hours, — attempting to make something out of essentially nothing. Finally, after what seemed like an eternity, I was done,— for now. Shatzi's little body may have looked like a patchwork quilt that missed out at the county fair, but she, none the less, was back together, — minus a few parts. The final step was the application of specialized jell pads over her injuries. These amazing pads absorbed discharge fluids from healing tissue, which in turn, aided the regrowth of healthy skin. It would be a very slow process, however, because so much skin was missing, and skin regeneration takes a long time, — only about 2mm per day. That's approximately 1/16 of an inch, — not much! Shatzi was hospitalized for several days, and continued to receive intravenous fluids, antibiotics and pain meds. Everyone realized it was going to be a long haul, but at least we were giving the little munchkin a fighting chance.

Over the next several months Shatzi endured countless bandage changes with minimal complaint, and it was exciting to monitor the skin regeneration and the healing progress. The treatments were working, albeit very slowly, but like the saying goes, wine just gets better with time. Shatzi was, without a doubt, one of my best patients, and she seemed to know that we were trying to help her. Throughout the whole ordeal, her gentle spirit never seemed to falter. However, — there were a few times, especially during those touchy bandage changing sessions, when she'd let me know that I'd crossed the line. She'd give me a dirty look with those dark little eyes of hers, along with a slight lip curl, as if to say, "Watch it buster!". I'd apologize profusely, and then we'd be friends again. In spite of it all, she really was a very patient and forgiving little girl.

In time, Shatzi's wounds healed much better than origionally hoped for, and hair even grew in and around some of the scar tissue. She was looking pretty good. She adapted to being a tripod without missing a beat, and wasn't about to let a missing hind leg cramp her style. Shatzi may have had a new look, but she was still a "little darling", and she made sure everybody knew it.

Amazing little "Shatzi"

The Plaque

One of the requirements of a prospective veterinary student was to spend 300 documented hours shadowing a veterinarian. The student would observe, up close and personal, all the aspects involved with being a veterinarian. The experience was often an eye opener for the students, and it gave them an opportunity to see if veterinary medicine really was their "cup of tea".

Sheryl was a pre-vet student at nearby Eastern Washington University. She'd grown up on a farm, had been around animals all her life, and wanted to become a veterinarian for as long as she could remember. She was doing well in school, had good grades, was an excellent communicator, and had that "it" factor of self confidence and determination. Sheryl was a beautiful young lady both inside and out. Not only did she have a strong working faith, but she had her priorities in the right place too. She would spend three weeks observing at the Medical Lake Veterinary Clinic, fulfilling a portion of the 300 hours required before applying to veterinary school. Sheryl observed patient examinations, diagnostic procedures and treatments, and even assisted on a few minor surgical procedures. She did great, and was very appreciative of being afforded the opportunity and experience.

Three weeks had past since Sheryl had completed her time with us, and I was pleasantly surprised when she walked through the clinic door that day. She was smiling, as usual, and carrying a package in her arms. "Doctor Roloff" she said, "I learned a lot during my time here, and I've made a little thank-you gift for you. Well, actually, I didn't make it all by myself, — my grandpa helped me." She then handed me the package with gleeful anticipation in her eyes. I carefully unwrapped the package, and found a beautiful wall plaque inside. The plaque was personalized with my name, and had "A Prayer for Animals" by Albert Schweitzer decoupaged upon it. I was familiar with that prayer and had read it before. I was, most definitely, moved by the thoughtful gift. You see, Albert Schweitzer was a person that I'd always respected and admired. He was a man of many talents, and what really impressed me about him was his profound reverence for life, — all life. I totally identified with that point of view. "Sheryl" I said, "this is one of the most meaningful gifts that I've ever received. Thank you so very much." I also told her that I'd hang the plaque in my office, — which I did.

Several days later, one of our staff members came into my office and noticed the plaque mounted on the wall. She paused momentarily, read the inscription, then turned to me and said, "That's very nice, — but who is Albert Scheitzer?" "You mean Albert Schweitzer." I replied. "No, — Albert Scheitzer. That's what it says here." She responded. I got up from my desk, and went over to take a closer look at the plaque. Sure enough, — whoever meticulously printed the prayer onto the plaque had unfortunately misspelled the name of the renown humanitarian and author. "You're right!" I said. "But you know what, — it's the thought that really counts and matters."

That beautiful plaque hung on my office wall for many years, and I frequently read that "Prayer for Animals". Those simple, yet eloquent words, often kept me focused on my purpose and calling to be a veterinarian.

The plaque

Who's Next

It was just one of those days, — a real head shaker. It all started with a 10 year old boy walking into the clinic, delicately clutching something in one of his mom's favorite kitchen towels. With a concerned look on his face, and compassion in his voice, he said, "I found an injured bird, — can you help it?" The young man was quickly ushered into exam room #1, where he gently place the towel and it's contents upon the exam table. Careful unwrapping of the towel revealed a young robin, — motionless, but still breathing, although ever so slightly. I asked the boy, "Where did you find the bird?" "By the window." He replied. "I heard something hit the window, and when I went to see what happened, — there it was, — just laying there, — is he going to die?" "I don't know yet." I answered. "He could, — he's definitely in trouble, — lots of things could be going on here, — a concussion, broken neck, a fractured wing. — He's in shock, and we need to address that first or else he'll surely die. — Sandy, — get the Rescue Remedy." Rescue Remedy is a special homeopathic preparation composed of flower essences that help an individual cope with various stressful conditions, including shock. I pried the robin's beak open with a small forceps, and deposited several drops of the concoction on the back of the limp robin's tongue. No more than 5 seconds or so had passed, when suddenly, the young bird began to move it's beak, blink his eyes, shake his head, and struggle to get free. I gave the little guy a couple more drops of the stuff, and that's all it took. It was like magic! That little bird went, at warp speed, from a state of being nearly dead to. — "Hey, get me out'ta here! — I've got things to do and people to see." He started flapping his wings, obviously not broken, and was getting pretty animated, so we placed him in a small, dark cardboard box so he could cool his jets for a while. You could hear him hopping around inside, and a quick peek into the box revealed that the little guy's bottom end was working pretty good too.

That little bird had certainly dodged a bullet, so to speak, and if that concerned young man hadn't been such a good Samaritan, — well, that little robin would've been history. I instructed the boy to take the robin back home and release the bird where he'd found it. All's well that ends well, and hopefully the bird had learned a lesson.

My next patient was a real cutie, — an eight week old Cockapoo puppy named "Tootsie". It was her first visit to the vet, but she didn't care, — all she seemed interested in was getting petted, scratched, and tickled. She also had, what seemed to be, the fastest tongue in the West. Heck, — she could lick your face in the blink of an eye, — you couldn't see it coming. Tootsie was a real charmer, — that was for sure. In fact, the entire staff took turns cuddling that little girl. Sandy, our office manager even took Tootsie along for a short ride around the clinic in her smock pocket. Well, — after everyone had gotten their "puppy fix" for the day, it was time to get down to business with the exam, vaccinations, and worming. Tootsie was a brave little trooper, didn't complain, and passed with flying colors.

It was about half an hour after Tootsie had gone home when Sandy asked, "Did one of our patients have an accident somewhere in the waiting room? I keep getting this "drift", and I'm not sure where it's coming from." Everyone started looking for the tell-tale evidence, but nothing was found, — in fact, nobody could detect any offending odor of any kind, anywhere, — but

Sandy could! In frustration, Sandy thrust her hand into her smock pockets, — "Ooh!–Oh no! – Oh gosh! – I found the source of the smell. — The puppy POOPED in my pocket and I've been carrying that thing around with me for the last hour. No wonder I could smell it and nobody else could. At least we've got a really fresh sample for a fecal analysis." It was one of those cherished moments where everyone came together and laughed until their sides ached. It felt good to laugh so hard. We seized the moment, — because each day in veterinary medicine was not unlike riding an emotional rollercoaster, — dealing with routine, to challenging, to catastrophic cases, punctuated by humorous interludes.

"Hey Doc, — are you ready for the next one? — This one should be interesting." Those kind of comments from our receptionist invariably set off streams of distorted mental images, — most of which never came to fruition, thank goodness. But what she said next would never have crossed my mind. "What'a we got?" I asked. "It's a garter snake that got attacked by their cat. It's got a nasty bite wound on it somewhere." She replied. "I want to see how you handle this one. — It should be really interesting."

It wasn't long before Carrie Dwyer came sashaying through the front door, clutching a small wicker basket that resembled the baskets used by the snake charmers in India. Carrie carefully removed the lid of the basket to reveal a little green snake and proudly said, "This is Theata, she's a three year old Garter Snake, and she's a good girl, — isn't she." That mini-serpent just sat there in a tight coil, peering up at her owner with it's tiny dark eyes, and rhythmically flicking it's forked tongue in and out. The little snake seemed oblivious to the gaping, one and a half inch long traumatic wound located midway on her back. "She'll need stitches won't she Doc." "Most definitely" I replied. "Can you hold her while I give her a local anesthetic?" Carrie nodded her head, yes, and then asked, "How many snakes have you worked on Doc?" "Not many, and suturing one up is a whole new ballgame for me, — but there's always a first for everything." Carrie giggled nervously.

The local anesthetic took effect almost immediately. Once the area was numb, I then cleaned and disinfected the tissue, applied an antibiotic solution, and selected a 4-0 vicryl suture for closure. The needle passed through the scales with ease, and that surprised me. I was expecting more resistence. Six interrupted (separate) sutures (stitches) were needed to close the wound, which came together very nicely. Carrie was pleased and pleasantly surprised, considering the way it looked initially. Theata flicked her tongue a few more times, coiled back up in the basket, and was ready to go home. As Carrie and Theata were about to leave the clinic, my last words of advice were, "Theata, you've got to stay away from that cat, or learn to move faster." She just stared back at me and flicked her tiny forked tongue in my direction.

The next case just showed up without an appointment. I was in my office, working on Patient records when Rachel, our receptionist, suddenly popped her head around the corner and chimed out, — "Oh Doc, there's someone here who wants to see you. He wants to show you something." I didn't expect to see Gene standing at the reception counter, and since he wasn't an animal owner, my initial thought was that he'd come to sell me a raffle ticket or get a donation for his service club. But then he stooped down, picked up a cardboard box, looked me straight in the eyes, smiled mischievously, and said, "Do you want a stray cat?" I told him, "Not at the moment, but let's see what'cha got here, — maybe we can find a good home for your new little friend." One of our missions at the veterinary clinic was to find nice homes for strays and unwanted cats and kittens. We usually had one or two kittens in an exercise pen placed in the waiting room, with a sign attached that read, "I'm available for adoption". We'd place about thirty to thirty-five cats and kittens each year. It was a win-win situation.

Gene was ushered into exam room #1, where he unceremoniously plopped the box on the exam table. "I found this thing hanging on the screen door this morning. I was going out to get the newspaper, — opened the door, — and there it was, — spread eagle, — hooked onto the screen door, — look'n me eyeball to eyeball." He then reached into the box and pulled out a small black tortoise shell colored kitten. "Isn't this the ugliest cat you've ever seen? Its mother must have abandoned it, — she probably thought that it was pretty ugly too, — and just kicked it out!" Gene and his wife, Carol, hadn't owned a pet for a long time, and I'd assumed they didn't want this one either. So, I told Gene, "Let me check this tiny "Cling-on" over, and see what we can do for her. Gene, we've definitely got a little girl here, and she's about seven weeks old, — probably recently weaned by the mom." She didn't have any fleas, her temp was normal, — no ear mites, heart and lungs sounded good, and her eyes and nose were nice and clean, — no drainage. "Gene"' I said, "This little girl isn't ugly! — She's actually pretty cute, — in her own special way. Tortoise shell colored kittens may look a bit unusual but the color pattern gets prettier over time. She'll become a very beautiful cat, — believe me. What we need to do now is vaccinate and deworm her so she can be adopted. We'll find her a good home in no time at all." After a momentary pause, Gene blurted out, "I'll take her home with me. — I'll see if I can find out where she came from." "Are you sure?" I asked. "Yeah", Gene replied. "Carol can help me." I reminded Gene that the kitten needed a booster vaccination in a month. — He nodded, and then took off on his humanitarian mission.

A month had passed, and as I peeked at the appointment schedule on that one particular morning, I noticed a kitten booster vaccination on the books, and recognized the phone number too. It was Gene's number, — "He must not have found the owner yet." I thought to myself. When the appointment time had arrived,

Gene wasn't alone, — Carol was accompanying him. They were all smiles, and acted like two high school kids who'd just snuck out of study hall. "We've decided to keep her." Gene said. Carol chimed in, "She's a good little girl, — you can't help but love her, — even though she isn't the prettiest cat in the neighborhood." Gene then said laughingly, "Yeah, we decided to name her "UGGY", — ya know, — short for ugly cat. Ugly Cat is a little to harsh a name, don't ya think?" Carol gazed down lovingly at "Uggy" as she gently stroked the kitten, and said, "We don't want to give our little girl a complex. — do we Uggy." I nodded in agreement, chuckled to myself, and continued on with the examination. I reassured Gene and Carol that tortoise shell colored cats are like fine wine, — they just get better and more beautiful with time. Such was the case with "Uggy". She'd indeed found the perfect home where she was a loved and pampered member of the family. Without a doubt, "Uggy" truly enriched Gene and Carol's lives in more ways than one.

"Uggy"

The ole saying, "different strokes for different folks" really hit the nail on the head with my next case. Autumn Steller was the independent, free thinking daughter of two hippies from the 60's. One's initial impression of her, by her "liberated" attire and easy-going demeanor, was "this is one very likeable, yet some-what eccentric individual". She wore her emotions on her sleeve, would unabashedly express her opinions about anything, whether you wanted to hear them or not, and was, to say the least, — very uninhibited, in a pleasant sort of way. Autumn was definitely one of a kind.

Autumn brought her four year old Shih Tzu, named "Emily" to the clinic for an eye exam. There was no hesitation with this woman, — she wasn't a kibitzer, and there was no beating around the bush with her. "Emily's eyes have been watering more lately. She gets gunk in the corners, — rubs them a lot more, and's been squinting more too, — What's going on?" I assured Autumn that I'd do my best to solve the problem, then started the exam. Emily was a sweet little girl, — gyrating her petite body all through the exam, — thinking it was all just fun and games. Emily was a head rubber, and she wasn't especially discerning about what she rubbed up against. It was an affectionate marking type of behavior that had inadvertently caused some problems. She'd rub her face on a person's clothing, on the floor, and on just about anything that was available. Too much of a good thing can usually lead to problems, and that was the case here. Emily's excessive face rubbing had irritated her eyes, — producing more tearing and eye discharge, — which resulted in more "gunk" accumulating in the corners of her eyes, —her long hair would stick to the gunk, — it was uncomfortable, — so Emily did what comes naturally, — she rubbed her eyes more. It was a vicious circle of events which resulted in a classic case of conjunctivitis and corneal edema. I trimmed back the long hair from around her eyes, cleaned and medicated them, and dispensed special eye drops to help relieve the itching, reduce the swelling, and combat any infections. She was also fitted with the proverbial "cone-of-shame" that needed to be worn for several days. While fitting Emily with the cone, I noticed something a little unusual, — she had a small earring in the lower part of her left ear. "Wow" I said, "When did she get this? I've never seen a dog with an earring before." "Oh, — I had that done a couple months ago, — took her in, — got her ear pierced, — and she didn't seem to mind at all. — I'm thinking about having the other ear done too. What do you think?" "Uh, — looks nice." I replied. "But watch out for infections and for it getting caught on things." Autumn shook her head, acknowledging that she understood, then gently picked up Emily, and affectionately said to her, "Oh, — you look so cute with your little earring and new collar." — I thought to myself, "Ah yes, — different strokes for different folks."

Such is the life of a veterinarian. — No two days were ever the same, — not many boring moments, — many challenges, — with people as well as the animals, but it sure made life very interesting and fun. That's why I loved it!

Q & A's

Veterinarians get asked oodles of questions, and some are obviously much easier to answer than others. Helping people to learn more about animals and their medical conditions was, and still is, very important to me. There were times when I was asked certain questions that required some honest soul searching before answering. Those occasions always prompted me to pause and reflect upon my experiences as a youth which eventually set me on the pathway to becoming a veterinarian.

Some of the most honest and straight forward questions come from the younger set. They don't beat around the bush, — being politically correct isn't in their vocabulary, — yet, and for the most part, they're very direct and uninhibited. Psalms 8:2 and Matthew 21:16 really nail it, — "Out of the mouths of babes".

Having my granddaughter visit the veterinary clinic was always a delight. It didn't seem to matter to her if I was in the exam room with a patient or not, she'd just wander in and belly up to the exam table, just like she owned the place. I'd quickly explain to the clients what was going on, and thankfully everyone just went with the flow and seemed to understanding the uinhibited intrusion. What was really amazing though was how the animals responded. They didn't seem to mind at all, in fact, they'd calm down somewhat, and some even started wagging their tails in delight at the sudden appearance of a little person. After the exams, my granddaughter often shadowed me into my office where I'd sit down to complete the patient medical records. It was then that the inquisition would begin. — "Papa Jim, why do you like taking care of animals?" "It's a long story, sweetie. It all started when I was about your age, — on the farm. The animals were my friends, — my closest friends, really. They were my playmates and companions. We were together all day long. — I'd talk to them, — they listened, — and seemed to understand too. We did all kinds of stuff together." "What kind of stuff, Papa?" — "Oh, I'd go with the barn cats and watch them hunt and catch mice. They were really good at it too." "Did they let you hold them, Papa Jim?" — Some of them did, but barn cats are usually pretty wild, skittish, and afraid of people. But I managed to tame a few of them down to where they trusted me enough to let me pet them and eventually hold them." "They liked you, huh?" "Yes Amy, — they did, and I liked them too."

"One time, when I was about 6 years old, I thought I'd take one of the barn kittens, sneak him into the house, and show him my room. It was cooler that day, so I stuffed the little guy inside my jacket and zipped it up tight. He liked it in there. It was dark, and cozy. He just snuggled up, laid there quietly, and I could feel the warmth of his little body. It was pretty neat. When I got up to the house, I was hoping that my mom was busy doing something, so that I could slip by without being noticed, — but that didn't happen. As I entered the front door, cradling and protecting the package in my coat, there she stood, — looking at me with those "All Knowing" eyes. "Jimmy, — what do you have in your jacket?" "Uh, — nothing," I quickly replied, and tried to not look guilty. "Then why are you holding your hands that way?" She asked. Panic started to flood in and I felt ashamed for not being truthful, so I thought I'd try to come up with a good answer. Suddenly a little grey furry head with two big wide opened eyes popped out the top of my jacket, — just under my chin. "What's that cat doing in my house?" Mother forcefully yelled. — "Get it out of here RIGHT NOW! You know better than that. — No cats are allowed in the house!" Mother's loud voice scared the poor little kitten out of its wits, and it suddenly jettisoned out from my jacket and immediately took off in the direction of the living room at warp speed. Mother was in hot pursuit with her dish towel flailing in the air. The panic-stricken kitten was desperately looking for an escape route, when it suddenly spotted the new set of drapes around the large living room window. The little guy went scratching and clawing up the right side of the drapes as fast as he could with mother yelling and swinging the dish towel at him. He made it to the top, unscathed, and then clumsily maneuvered across the cornice to the other side, then shinnied down the other side of the drapes, and took off in the direction of my room. I eventually caught my frightened little friend and took him back to the safety of the barn. His poor little heart was really a pounding.

Well, — mother's new drapes got initiated and didn't look quite as nice as they once did, — I got reintroduced to the "board of education". "What's that, Papa Jim?" "It's a very memorable spanking, Sweetie." I said. "The kind that lingers for a long time, and one that leaves no doubt about what is acceptable and what is not. That was the last time I ever tried to sneak a barn cat into the house. The kitten eventually forgave me and we were friends again."

"What other animals did you have around the farm when you were growing up?" — "Oh, we had dogs, cows, pigs, chickens, a few rabbits, a couple sheep, and that's about it. — Once in a while a porcupine would show up, and there were a few raccoons, skunks, coyotes, and badgers that wandered in now and then. But one of the neatest little animals I came across was the horned toad. I'd find them out in the fields. They were hard to see because the color of their little bodies was about the same color as dirt, and they were shaped like small dirt clods, and could move pretty fast if they wanted to. They looked kind of prehistoric, but they were gentle little creatures and easy to handle when caught. I really liked those little guys."

"What kind of dogs did you have, Papa Jim?" "Oh Sweetie, — I had lots of dogs when I was growing up. My dad, your great grandpa, was a real dog magnet. People would just give him dogs all the time, and he'd bring them home. Let's see, — over the years, I had a Collie, several Collie mixes, a Schnauzer, a Cocker Spaniel, a Springer Spaniel, an Australian Shepherd, some Heinz-57 types, and a Chihuahua." "That's a lot, Papa. Why'd you have so many?" "It's a sad story, Sweetie. You see,—, your great grandpa didn't really understand how important it was for dogs to be vaccinated, and I unfortunately had to watch many of my best friends die from a very bad disease called distemper. That was really tough. I desperately wanted to help my friends, and keep them from dying like that. That's when I decided to become an animal doctor, a veterinarian, Eventually I found out about vaccinating dogs and how those shots could keep them from getting distemper and other bad stuff. I finally convinced your great grandpa to vaccinate the dogs, and you know what." "What" "None of our dogs ever died from distemper after that. Now you see why it's so important to keep your dog current on its vaccinations." "But I don't have a dog, Papa Jim.". "Someday you will Sweetie, — someday you will."

The chickens were kind of special too, — they were my first audience. I'd go into the chicken coup, and there where about 100 chickens sitting on their perches, — just chillin' out. I'd set up a wooden apple box on its end and start preaching to them. They'd just sit there, quietly clucking and looking at me with one eye, trying to figure out what was going on. I had their attention, and I relished in the moment. — they seemed like they completely understood what I was saying to them. It was great! — It was a real confidence booster. I always felt sorry for the one little chick who was being bullied and picked on. Sometimes it got so bad that the poor chick started to bleed from all the cruel pecking. When that happened, we'd get some "Mrs. White's Bluing" and put it on the bloody spots. That blue coloring seemed to stop all the pecking, — it worked like magic! — I really liked the chickens." "That's good that you helped the chickens, Papa Jim." "Thanks Sweetie."

"Did you always like the animals, Papa Jim?" "Yeah," — even the wild ones. I'll never forget the coyote incident." "You had a coyote Papa?" "No, — not really, but there was one particular encounter that I'll always remember. It was very early in the morning when, — all of a sudden, — the chickens started squawking like crazy. Chickens don't panic like that unless something is definitely wrong. Their loud warning cackles woke up everybody in the house. Your great grandpa yelled out to me, "Coyote! — Jimmy, — get the gun and shoot that thing before it gets all the chickens." I leaped out of bed, — wide awake, heart pounding, — got my shoes and jeans on in record time, — grabbed the 30-30 rifle, and headed out of the house to "get" the threatening intruder. I was a really good shoot, — very accurate, and hit my target almost all the time. Farm boys were taught early in life about guns, how to shoot, and how to kill what you aimed at. It was sort of a right of passage, and I excelled at it, — I was good, — real good, — and confident! When I got out by the chicken barn, — all the squawking suddenly stopped, but the chickens still milled around, acting worried and uneasy, — there was something still out there. I froze in my tracks, — motionless, — letting my eyes adjust to the predawn light against the beige colored fields, — hoping to spot my target. It was so very still and quite, — I slowed my breathing so as to more easily hear any movement. I could almost hear and feel my own heart beating, — it was so quiet. I FELT him, — I couldn't see him, — but I KNEW he was there. I didn't want to make a move, — and blow my cover, — he would have to show himself, and when he did, I'd get him! Somehow I sensed that he was in front of me, but I couldn't see anything, — and he knew that too. Neither of us wanted to make a move, — it was a waiting game. I was facing East, and with the rising morning sun, only a few minutes away, if the coyote was really there in front of me, as I sensed he was, — well, — his silhouette would slowly be revealed, and I'd have an easy shot. Time seemed to stand still, — standing there motionless, waiting for my chance. Gradually the first rays of the morning sun began to peek above the horizon, casting a pinkish hue over the ground. My heart started pounding in anticipation of seeing my target, — then, slowly but surely, the silhouette of the coyote came into view. It sort of materialized out of nothing. I couldn't believe it, — he was just standing there, — only about 20 feet in front of me, —with his left side exposed, — I had a clean heart shot, — and as I took careful aim, he just stood there like a statue, — using his survival skills of remaining totally motionless and invisible. He was a beautiful creature, — young, strong, and cleaver, but I had him directly in my sights. I paused and thought about how the two of us tried to outsmart each other, and I truly believed, or choose to believe, that there was a mutual respect between us. I couldn't shoot this guy, —he deserved a chance to live. So, — I moved my sights a few feet over his back and squeezed the trigger. The load crack of the rifle and the sound of the bullet whistling through the air sent the coyote running off at lightning fast speed, leaving only a cloud of dust hanging in the still morning air. "Goodbye little buddy, have a good life, and be careful." I said to myself as he disappeared out of sight.

"When I went back into the house, your great grandpa called out to me, "Did you get him?" I told him that it was too dark, — that I didn't have a good look at the coyote, and that I flat out missed the shot. I never did tell him what really happened, but I always felt good about sparing that beautiful animal's life. The whole experience of matching wits with a very crafty and perceptive wild animal, and choosing to let it live, was neat. That simple act of compassion fueled a desire deep within me to save more animals' lives, and believe or not, that coyote incident actually helped convince me to become a veterinarian."

"Papa Jim, — did you ever get bit?" "Oh yes, Sweetie, — many times, — and not only did I get bit, but I got scratched, stepped on, kicked, horn whipped, pooped and peed on more times than I can remember too, — not fun, — but part of the job." "Did you get hurt?" "Sometimes, — I've had more than my share of bruises, and I've also had to get stitched up a few times, and believe me, — I've got quite a few battle scars. But you know what?" "What?" "I still love helping animals, and for the most part, they seem to know that too. There's kind of an unspoken understanding between us, — pretty neat, huh."

One of the most frequently asked series of questions at the veterinary clinic was, "Isn't it hard to put an animal down? How can you do that? I couldn't do that." Those were heartfelt questions that required honest and soul searching answers. I usually replied by saying something like, "Yes, — it can be hard, — it's never easy. It is often a very emotional time for everyone present, because that animal is, in most cases, a very special friend and a beloved member of the family. I love animals too, and when their quality of life has come to an end, I'm there to humanely relieve their pain and suffering, and help them cross over quickly and painlessly, with dignity and respect. I see it as an act of loving kindness, and most people agree with that and are very appreciative. It's always a bitter-sweet time. — It always makes my heart hurt, but I can take consolation in knowing that I've helped the animal and the owners through a very difficult time."

When asked about my early exposure with animals, — nothing could top the "cow with the balloon" incident. I was a very adventurous and inquisitive little 5 year old farm boy who spent a lot of time exploring the out buildings, climbing in and on farm machinery, and most importantly of all, spending quality time with the animals. During one of my visits to the cow barn, I saw something that stopped me dead in my tracks. There, – standing right in front of me, was a cow with a big pink balloon under her outstretched tail! "WOW"! I muttered to myself. I'd never seen anything like that before. I was bewildered and filled with excitement, – all at the same time, and when that happens, – go tell mom. I ran as fast as I could back to the house, barged through the kitchen door, and even though out of breath, I blurted out, "MOM, there's a cow in the barn with a pink balloon under her tail"! Mother quickly whirled around from the sink where she was washing dishes, and sternly said to me, "Jimmy, – you stay right here in the house. – Leave that cow alone! Don't bother her. – I'll tell dad all about it when he comes in from the field." That wasn't the answer I'd expected. I felt disappointed because I thought she'd be as excited as I was, but she wasn't. I waited few minutes, but curiosity got the best of me. So, I snuck out of the house, went back down to the barn, and witnessed the miraculous birth of a calf. An experience that I'll never forget and one which helped shape my future.

Ear – atations!

Ears are sort of the Rodney Dangerfields of anatomical structures. – They just don't get any respect, – are underappreciated, and often overlooked. Those unique sound receivers come in a variety of sizes and shapes, but one thing they all have in common is their basic design, – a thin sheet of cartilage, to provide form and shape, sandwiched between two layers of highly vascularized skin. They're essentially just sitting out there, somewhat vulnerable to injury, – and when problems occur, they're usually biggies, – both literally and figuratively speaking.

"Good morning everybody!" I merrily chimed out upon entering the clinic that Monday morning. "What's on tap today? Anything interesting and exciting?" "Pretty much routine stuff most of the morning." Angela, our receptionist, relayed from the front desk. "A cat neuter, – an OVH (ovariohysterectomy/spay) on a dog, – some vaccinations, – and a dog with a swollen ear." "Whose first?" I asked. "Sally Gates is dropping off Jessie, on her way to work. Jessie's been shaking her head a lot lately, and now her ear is all puffed up. – Sally says it looks kind of like a little pillow." "Those things don't just develop out of nowhere." I interjected. "We've got to check her ears for what might be causing all the head shaking."

The clinic door suddenly swung open and Jessie, a six year old Golden Retriever, came prancing, unabashedly, into the waiting room with owner, Sally Gates, in tow. Jessie whimpered with excitement, even though she was obviously hurting, as evidenced by her head being tilted sharply to the right. Jessie would occasionally paw at her right ear and shake her head violently, but her desire to play "scratch & tickle" took precedence over her pain and discomfort". Jessie was a good girl. A little on the pudgy side, but still a joy to have as a patient. Sally kept entreating Jessie to "settle down!" as the two of them sashayed into the 2nd exam room. Without hesitation Sally said, "Look at that ear, Doc. That's not right! It's all swollen. Do what you have to do, and give me a call at work. I've got to get going, – I'm late already." She quickly signed the release forms, – said that Jessie hadn't eaten breakfast, – and was out through the door in a flash. "Well Jessie," I said. "Let's see what we can do for you."

It was glaringly obvious. – Jessie had an ear hematoma, and that's why her ear looked like a mini-water balloon, – but instead of it being filled with good ole water, – it was filled with stagnant blood and blood clots. All the head shaking and pawing at the ear had damaged some of the vessels in the ear. The blood then leaked out of the vessels, – organized, and clotted in the area between the skin and the cartilage of her injured ear. – and that's what produced the swelling. It can be a tricky proposition to treat and get an ear hematoma to properly heal without scarring complications and major disfigurement. Many surgical procedure options for ear hematomas were out there, but I'd had good success with minimal complications using the cannula method, – and that's the approach I chose to use with Jessie.

We placed Jessie under a general anesthetic, and when she was sleeping comfortably, the work began. After shaving, cleaning, and prepping her ear, an incision was made directly into the pinna of the ear in order to remove the blood clots, fibrin, and stagnant blood. Following a thorough cleaning of the now empty cavity, a cannula was inserted into the tip of the ear to provide drainage during the healing process, while the internal tissue was reattaching.

The next thing to do was to scope the ear canal and look for what may have caused Jessie discomfort and initiated all that head shaking. – There it was!! – a big hunkin foxtail, – way down there, – rubbing on Jessie's eardrum. I carefully removed the culprit with a long forceps, cleaned the ear canal of excessive moisture and debris, and instilled some medication. Then I told her, "There you go Jessie. – That ole bugger's outa there. – Your ear's all fixed up, – and now you should feel a whole lot better. – We're done."

Jessie was transferred to a nice warm and quiet recovery cage where she could slowly wake up without any distractions. It was now time to call Sally and give her an update. "Hi Sally, – Doc here. We're all done." "What did you find, Doc?" "Several things." I replied. "She had an ear hematoma, – sort of a huge blood blister in the ear. Blood vessels most likely broke inside the flap of her ear when she shook her head so hard, – and all that intense pawing at the ear didn't help matters either. I removed a lot of stuff outa there and put a drain in the end of the ear flap. We'll leave the drain in there for a couple weeks to assist healing. I also scoped her ears and found what may have started the whole thing. She had a big cheat grass awn (foxtail awn) irritating the eardrum, plus there was an excessive amount of moisture in her ear canal." "Oh Doc, "Sally interjected "I think I know how that happened. We went to the lake cabin last weekend. She just loves it there. – She's in and out of the lake all day long, and has the time of her life, – chasing birds and squirrels in all the underbrush. I betcha that's when she got that stuff in her ears." "I think you're right, Sally. Next time, – wipe out the ears and use some ear drying solution whenever she goes swimming. That should help with that moisture issue, but dealing with those foxtails is a whole different matter.

Jessie recovered nicely, with minimal tissue scarring and disfigurement of her ear. Sally did her best to prevent recurrences,

– but foxtails and excessive water in the ear canal are never ending challenges to deal with, – are always sources of, – "Ear-atations" and have the potential to lead to bigger problems as well, – like the dreaded ear hematomas.

What? -Me Worry?

The face of a whimsical, fictitious individual named Alfred E. Newman graced almost every issue of MAD Magazine. His goofy expression, – sort of carefree and clueless, was always accompanied by the caption, "What? – Me Worry?" Looking at that guy couldn't help but make a person smile and realize that life's challenges were highly over rated and really weren't that big of a deal. One of my patients, a six year old black Labrador Retriever named "Bear" seemed to embody Alfred E. Newman's philosophy about life.

It never ceases to amaze me how fate often steps in and causes people's lives to cross after many years of separation. Thirty years had come and gone since I'd last seen Ray Jehry at his father's small general store in Ralston, Washington. A rural hamlet of about twenty-five citizens, a church, two grain elevators, a railroad station, small park, and a quaint little general store with a tiny post office located in the back, next to the cooler. The rough and worn wooden slat floor would creak as you walked across it. Neatly stocked shelves from floor to ceiling, adorned the walls. Items were even displayed in half cut wooden barrels, and the wonderful smell of "Dixie-Cups" filled the air. It was a magical place, and I loved going in there, – All those great memories came rushing in from my memory bank when Ray came walking into the clinic with Bear shuffling along at his side. It was like "ole home week", but our reminiscing was short-lived because

Bear was hurtin, and obviously needed some major help with his mobility issues.

"What's goin on with Bear?" I asked. "He's been having trouble walking, – has a hard time getting up and down, – limps a lot more, – doesn't want to play." Ray replied. There was a tone of sorrowful resignation in his voice. "Ray" I responded. "let's see what we've got going on here." After examining Bear, I told Ray that Bear was showing a limited range of motion in his hind legs and was shuffling way more than normal. His hips were painful on palpation, and there was abnormal wear on the tops of the nails on his rear paws, – indicating that Bear was dragging his paws because pain was restricting free movement and inhibiting proper paw placement. I also pointed out that Bear's hip and rear leg muscles were atrophied and weakened due to reduced usage, plus he walked with his head down and was shifting his body weight more forward in order to lessen the load on his rear end. "Ray", I said. "All the signs are pointing to hip dysplasia or major arthritis of the hip joints, – but we need to take x-rays to confirm it."

Bear was given a general anesthetic so he could go through the x-ray procedure without experiencing any discomfort. Bear was a pretty good sized boy, – about 85 pounds, and it took a little effort to get his relaxed body into the proper position for taking the x-rays. His hips were really tight, – preventing his hind legs from being fully extended, – not a good sign. We got the shots we needed, – developed the films, and then placed them up on the viewer. "WOW!" Both hips joints were severely dysplastic, and deformed, with extensive arthritic changes present all over the place. It was BAD! The worst hip dysplasia case that I'd ever seen. Those damaged hips had to be extremely painful to Bear, and it was a minor miracle that he could even walk, – period! His high pain threshold and determined "will" were about the only things enabling him to marginally cope with all the discomfort. You couldn't help but feel sorry for the guy.

I called his owner back to take a look at the x-rays, – so he could see for himself the severity of Bear's condition. First, – I showed Ray an x-ray of another dog whose hips were normal, then I flipped up Bear's x-rays. "YIKES!" Ray said with a tone of concern in his voice. "That doesn't look good. – Can anything be done for him, – or would it be better to put him out of his misery?" "Ray," I said, "putting Bear down isn't an option because there are a couple of good surgical procedures that could help him a lot. One involves total hip replacements, – pretty pricey, – and the other is what's called an excision arthroplasty, or another name for it is a femoral head osteotomy. That's where the painful arthritic head of the femur bone is surgically removed and then the body develops or produces a false joint, – no more painful rubbing. The down side is that it takes about 4 weeks for the patient to start using the leg again, – but after that, there's minimal to no pain, – it doesn't cost as much as the hip replacements, and the end results are usually quite good. Once the dog starts gaining strength in that leg, then the same surgical procedure can be done on the other hip." I think Bear would do well with the the femoral head osteotomy, – but you've got to be patient with his recovery time. It will take a while, but Bear is a good boy with a great attitude, – that's a key ingredient to the success of a surgery like this." It didn't take Ray very long to decide what he wanted to do. "Doc, – let's go with that cutting off the bone thing, – I'm not interested in no hip replacements. Can you do it Doc, or do I have to take him somewhere else?" "I can do it for you, Ray". "I replied. "So, – let's take a look at the schedule and set up a surgery time, – the sooner, the better."

On surgery day, – Bear came gimping into the clinic with a "laissez faire" demeanor, sporting that "What? – Me Worry?"

happy-go-lucky, clueless attitude, – hey, – "No worries mate." He had no idea of what was in store for him, – and that was probably a good thing. Bear was given a pre-anesthetic injection, and when he was nice and relaxed, the general anesthetic was administered. When he was comfortable in "La-La" land, the work started. Bear's entire left hip area was shaved, prepped, and draped for surgery. A six inch incision was then made over the top of the hip, – exposing the underlying muscles, – which were delicately transected at their attachment to the femur bone. Reflecting the now freed muscles dorsally allowed the hip joint to come into view, – and a small incision through the joint capsule provided excellent exposure to the inside of the joint. The problem area was now clearly visible. –WHAT A MESS!!! There were severe arthritic changes resembling mini boney stalagmites all over the place inside that joint. The x-rays looked bad, – but seeing it up close and personal was a whole different matter. It was a minor miracle that Bear could stand, – let alone put any weight on that leg and walk. Not only did it look awful, – Bear HAD to be experiencing a lot of pain and discomfort from all that stuff rubbing around in that joint. Well, – now we were about to remedy that for the ole boy. I proceeded to saw off the head and neck of the femur bone, and once that was done, I carefully smoothed off the remaining bone. The surgery had gone well, – it looked good, – and it was now time to put everything back together. First, I closed the joint capsule, – and then proceeded to reattach the muscles. The final step was to close the skin incision. –DONE! Bear was given antibiotic, and anti-inflammatory injections along with medications for pain before transporting him to recovery. We monitored Bear's recovery the rest of the day, and when I checked him later that evening, he was resting comfortably.

As I entered the clinic the following morning, I was greeted by the loud "thumping" sound of Bear's "Happy Tail" banging against the walls of his recovery cage. When he saw me, he maneuvered himself to a standing position, – all the while wagging his tail, and vocalizing, as if saying, "Hey, – get me something to eat, – and get me outta here!" When I walked over to his cage and asked him, "How you feelin this morning?". He wiggled his body all over the place, – thumped his tail even harder, and delicately touched the toes of his surgery leg to the floor. His appetite sure wasn't affected by the surgery because he devoured his bowl of food as if he'd been on a 40 day fast. "Hey Bear," I asked, "You want to go outside?" There went the tail again, – gads, – he could lay a serious leg whipping on somebody with that thing! I got one of the veterinary techs to help me manage this guy, because he was a handful of "Happy". We used a tummy sling on Bear to provide some stability, and took him outside for a short walk so that he could do his "business". Believe me, – all systems worked perfectly, – a "big" success! While on his "relief" walk, I noticed him attempting to place some weight on the surgery leg. "Bear", I chided, "you've got to take it easy on that leg for a while. You've gone through a major remodel job, and it'll take some time before you can use that thing again. Bear just looked at me with that Alfred E. Newman, "WHAT? ME WORRY?" expression on his face. I thought to myself, "This guy is going to be a handful to manage.

Before sending Bear home that afternoon, I reminded his owner about what to anticipate during the recovery period following an excision arthroplasty/femoral head osteotomy surgery. "Ray, – don't expect Bear to use that leg for at least 3-4 weeks. It takes time for the body to form a false joint of scar tissue. We can probably schedule the same surgery on the other hip in a few months. Just as I finished giving Ray my spiel, – down the hallway came our veterinary technician with Bear in tow. Ray and I instantly stopped talking and just stood there with that "dead fish" look on our faces, – eyes and mouths wide open. Bear wasn't hopping on three legs, – he was actually placing full weight, albeit lightly, on the surgery leg. "Hey Doc," Ray said sarcastically, "that was sure a short month, wasn't it!" "Wow!" I replied, "I thought Bear had a high pain threshold, – but this surprises me, – we still want him to have controlled activity for that first month." Ray just smiled, – tapped me on the shoulder and said, "Right!"

Bear was something else! He walked without a limp at the end of the first week, and was running on that leg seven days after that, – way ahead of what would normally be expected. On his one month post-op exam, Bear didn't limp into the clinic, – heck, – he bounded through the door, jumped around, and beat everybody's legs with his "happy tail". He was definitely feeling gooooood, – with no signs of discomfort whatsoever. It was great to see. "Ray", I commented, "You know you've got a very special guy here, don't ya." "Yeah" Ray replied, "He acts like his old self again. Runs all over the place, plays ball, – gets into things, – just acts goofy."

Bear's quality of life had drastically improved. Ray decided not to have the surgery done on Bear's right hip because, in Ray's own words, "Bear's great, – acts like nothing happened, – he's enjoying life, – I don't think he needs to go through another surgery and he never did.

Just Plain Weird

W ild and weird stories never cease to amaze, fascinate, and mystify people. Hearing or reading about those unusual accounts is one thing, but actually dealing with odd and unexpected stuff, up close and personal, is a whole different matter.

"Frankenkitty"

Case in point, – the "odd smelling" cat. I recall a lady calling the clinic and passionately telling our receptionist, "My cat smells bad, – real bad. He's eating O.K., –doesn't act sick, – but he just stinks. Is it his food? – Does he need a bath or something to make him smell better? Our receptionist told the lady, Taryn Reedy, that a lot of things could cause a cat to smell bad, – so, – the cat needed to be examined to find out what was causing the problem.

When Mrs. Reedy entered the clinic, the putrid odor emanating from the pet carrier she was toting, brutally heralded Morris's arrival. He was a neutered, two year old, orange and white classic tabby. A nice little guy, – and according to Mrs. Reedy, – he was her five year old daughter's favorite cat and playmate. "Those two are always together." Mrs. Reedy said. "That cat is really patient with her. He lets her do just about anything to him. –She's put bows on his head and has even tried to dress him up in some doll clothes. – He just goes along with it. Morris is definitely my daughter's cat." Morris was quickly ushered into the first exam room, the exhaust fans were immediately flipped on, and air freshener was liberally sprayed, – everywhere. It didn't take long to spot Morris's problem. He had a heavily matted section of hair, about two inches wide, and it extended all the way around his neck. It appeared to be firmly attached, moist, and smelled. I told Mrs. Reedy that Morris needed to be sedated so that the matted hair could be removed without pain and the area treated. She agreed.

When the little guy was snoozing comfortably, the arduous cleaning up process began. It was definitely an exercise in patience because the dense matt of hair was tightly affixed to the skin. Slowly but surely the mess was freed up, allowing the swollen, inflamed skin underneath the gooey, smelly matt to come into view. – it wasn't a pretty sight! After thoroughly cleaning away all the tacky serum and sloughed off necrotic (dead) skin and tissue, a very distinct, raw, red, angry looking line came into view. It went all the way around Morris's neck. While examining the wound, I noticed something that looked like a piece of metal embedded deep within the inflamed tissue. I grabbed a couple of forceps, spread the swollen tissue for a closer look, – and sure enough, – there it was, – no doubt about it, – a piece of metal that looked like a clasp of some sort. I managed to grasp the object, and applied gentle traction. It was firmly anchored, but I was able to move it slightly, and noticed that the little piece of metal was attached to what appeared to be a red colored piece of, – rubber. Bingo!!! I knew what it was! "You know what we've got here Rachel?" I said to my vet assistant. "No, – what is it Doc?" She replied. "Did you ever put your hair up in pigtails or in a ponytail, and used that little rubber band thing to hold your hair in place?" I asked. "Yeah. – Lots of times." "Well, – that's what we've got here, – and it's worked itself way down in there, – real good!" "How are you planning to remove it, Doc?" Rachel asked. "It looks like I'll have to cut it out, because there's extensive tissue reaction around it, and it won't move. – It's stuck in there. The problem with a rubber band around an appendage or the neck, as in this case, is that it continues to put constricting pressure on the skin and tissue. The steady compression of the rubber band cuts off blood supply to the points of contact, – the tissue dies, – there's secondary inflammation and some bleeding and release of serum, – it gets infected, – it starts smelling, – the body attempts to wall off the area with fibrous tissue, – and the process continues until the rubber band is removed. Now, – removing an embedded rubber band can be a little tricky. It can't just be pulled out. So, the only recourse is to cut it out, – and that's exactly what we have to do in this case."

The initial incision went all the way around Morris's neck, – much of the fibrous tissue, along with the offending rubber band, was dissected out and removed, and several layers of sutures (stitches) were needed to put Morris back together. The surgery was a complete success, but with stitches extending all the way around Morris's shaved neck, – he now looked like a little "FrankenKITTY".

I telephoned Mrs. Reedy to fill her in on what was found, and forewarned her about Morris's new look. She was concerned, but not surprised, and promised to have a little chat with her daughter about the do's and don'ts when playing dress-up with Morris.

"Filleted"

Kyle Murphy was partial to Irish Setters for a variety of reasons. He liked their color, the way they moved so gracefully and how their long, beautiful, silky hair flowed in the air as they ran. Their boundless energy, regal demeanor, and unconditional devotion also appealed to him. No doubt about it, – Mr. Murphy was an Irishman to the core, and that's another reason why he liked Irish Setters so much, – they were, – of course, – Irish. Although Irish Setters have a long and storied history of being outstanding hunting dogs, Kyle never hunted with his dogs. He wasn't a hunter, but he thoroughly enjoyed watching his two year old Irish Setter named "Danny" run wild and free through open fields in hot pursuit of anything that moved. They had fun, – most of the time, – but, – as we all know, – sometimes stuff just happens.

There was a field laying fallow nearby, about three miles out of town, that'd been allowed to revert back to its natural state. It was covered in native grasses, weeds, and some small bushes, – great cover for birds and all kinds of wildlife, – lots of interesting stuff for a dog to explore. Next to the open field stood the remnants of an old homestead, complete with aging trees, dilapidated out-buildings, a leaning windmill that'd seen better days, and some old, rusty farm machinery engulfed by Mother Nature. This was a great place for Danny to "let er go" and have some fun.

It was during one of their trips to the farm that fate stepped in and spoiled the day. Danny was out there, running around like crazy near the old homestead, – when suddenly he let out a pain-ful sounding "yip". Kyle instantly sensed that something had gone wrong, and he quickly yelled out, "DANNY, – COME! – DANNY!" It wasn't but a few seconds before Danny appeared, – blood all over his chest and front legs. It didn't look good! Kyle whisked Danny into his arms, – gently placed him in the front seat of the pickup, – and made a beeline for the veterinary clinic.

Danny and Kyle entered the clinic unannounced. Danny was subdued and sort of shuffled along, – seemingly oblivious to hav-ing the right side of his bloody chest hanging down and out of place, – but Kyle, on the other hand, was on the verge of losing it. The blood covered pair was quickly ushered into the exam room. Although the active bleeding had subsided, there was still some minor passive hemorrhaging. I immediately started my triage and assessment of Danny's condition, while simultaneously asking Kyle, "Tell me what's going on here. – How'd this happen? – Did you see it happen?" Kyle took a deep breath, – composed himself,

– and told me what he knew, – which wasn't much. While examining Danny's chest, I found that the skin and muscles attached to the right side of his chest had been cleanly, – almost surgically separated from his ribcage. It looked as if he'd been skillfully filleted, – neatly exposing his ivory colored ribs. Danny had to have run into something pretty sharp in order to inflict that type of wound. I explained the severity of the injury to Kyle, and told him about the challenges of reconstructing the laceration. "Kyle." I said. "I'm going to put Danny under with a general anesthetic, clean him up, and do my thing. So, while I'm doing that, why don't you go back out there, – look around, – and see if you can find something that Danny might have run into.

Danny went out like a light, – which was good, because that allowed me to get in there quickly to assess the extent of his injuries. It didn't take long to see that putting him back together wouldn't be easy. There wasn't much to reattach the severed muscles to. – But, before tackling that, all the blood soaked hair had to be shaved off and the wound thoroughly cleaned and prepped before beginning the reconstruction process. What a MESS!!! The wound extended from the 3rd to the 7th rib, and half way up the right side of Danny's chest. The only surgical option was to reattach the underside of the detached muscles to the intercostal muscles (the muscles between the individual ribs). It was a long, tricky and tedious procedure, – lots of carefully placed sutures (stitches) were needed to put Danny back together, – but eventually, as good ole "Larry the Cable Guy" would say, – "We Gotter Done!". Some post-op antibiotics and pain meds were given, and a fancy chest wrap using white elastic bandage tape with blue paw prints all over it was applied before placing Danny in a warm recovery cage. He did great!

Kyle stopped by the clinic several hours later to check on Danny, and told us what he'd found that could've been the culprit.

369

"Doc, there's an old farm implement out there with some big metal saucer-like parts on it. It's just sitting there, half hidden in the long grass and weeds. It looks pretty wicked!" "Kyle," I said. "Sounds like an old disc plow, and those saucer-like things you saw are actually the blades. They're curve shaped and have sharp edges too. That could be it! Danny could have run into one of those things, – and if he hit one of those sharp curved discs at just the right angle, – he'd fillet himself pretty good, – which is what probably happened. That explains it, – mystery solved."

Danny didn't appreciate having his activity restricted for a couple weeks, but it was necessary to ensure proper healing. In the end, Danny healed up nicely, and Kyle wisely chose a new, more open, and safer place to take Danny out for a run.

"Lost And Found"

Having a large, open, unfinished (second story) at the veterinary clinic was very handy, – lots of storage room. That's where years of patient files and boxes of past office paperwork found a home. It was an ideal place to store veterinary supplies, plus there was enough space for a "break-room" area, – complete with a TV, refrigerator, coffee maker, comfy chairs, and a futon. A nice getaway place for the staff that doubled as a home for a couple rescued cats, – Emma and Willow. They were nice cats, but they had some issues, – hiding issues.

It became second nature to check on those two each time one of us went upstairs for something or other. On one particular afternoon I saw Emma scurrying about, but Willow was conspicuously absent,– and she didn't respond when her name was called. I just assumed that she was hiding or fast asleep somewhere in an empty box or comfy hidey hole. "No big deal!" I thought to myself. But, when she didn't show up the next morning, – now,– that really started to concern me. I quickly briefed the entire staff about the problem, and asked everyone to go upstairs, as often as possible, and search the place, – from top to bottom. Willow was most likely trapped somewhere, and needed to be found, – PDQ!

It was later that afternoon, while completing a patient's chart in exam room #1, when I heard a muffled sound that resembled a faint, "meow". I instantly stopped what I was doing, – and listened intently for another sound, – nothing! I went back to my work, and then, a few minutes later, – there it was again. My first inclination was that the sound was coming from the air vent. So, I got a ladder, climbed up close to the vent and called out, – "Willow," – nothing. I put the ladder back into storage, returned to the exam room, – and suddenly, – I heard that muffled "meow" again, – but this time it seemed to be emanating from the electrical wall outlet next to the exam table. I grabbed my trusty stethoscope, – got down on my hands and knees, and started listening to the wall. At that very untimely moment, Angela, one of our veterinary assistants, walked into the room, – saw me crouched down in that compromised position, and laughingly asked, "Hey Doc, -whatcha doin down there? – You know, – that looks a little weird, – listening to a wall." "I know." I sheepishly replied. "But I think Willow is trapped in here. Let's check upstairs and look for an opening in the wall framing where she might have fallen into." Sure enough!!! There was a place where the carpenters hadn't finished closing off the wall framing, leaving a space about 4 inches by 16 inches between two wall studs, – not very big, – but neither was Willow. I grabbed a small mirror and a flashlight, and with a little maneuvering, managed to get a look down inside the wall. At first I couldn't see anything, but with a few minor adjustments of the light beam and mirror, – I saw some movement, – way down there. I ran downstairs and told everybody, "I found her, – she's in the wall." "What?– No way!– Really?"– Was the response I got. Now came the tricky part, – getting her out of there, – safely.

It was a crazy scene. Once again I got out my stethoscope, – listened to the wall so as to pinpoint Willow's exact location, – then located the positions of the wooden studs, – took a few measurements, – and drilled the pilot holes. Just as I began sawing through the wallboard, Angela came in the room and told me that the 3:40 appointment had arrived, and asked, "What should I tell her, Doc?" "Tell her that I'll be with her in a few minutes. I've got to clean up some of this mess first." I replied. When the client walked into the exam room with her cat, she smiled and delicately said, "I see you're doing a little remodeling today, Doc. I didn't know that you were also a carpenter." "Oh yeah, – I'm a man of many hidden talents." I replied. "Actually, I'm attempting to remove one of our clinic cats that's stuck inside the wall. She found an open space in the wall upstairs, -managed to climb in there, – and slipped down here." I received some raised eyebrows, a couple "Oh mys" and a few chuckles, then finished up the appointment and returned to my rescue mission. That scenario was repeated several more times, but eventually all the cuts in the sheetrock were made, and it was time to free Willow from her dark and dusty inner sanctum. Finally, – when the cut section of sheetrock was gently removed, – there she sat, – rather nonchalantly with a disgruntled expression on her face, – and covered in white sheetrock dust from head to toe. "Willow, – how you doin sweetheart?". I asked. She blinked several times and then emitted a soft, timid sounding, "meow". All was forgiven. A brief physical exam revealed that the extent of her injuries was limited to only a bruised ego. Willow was a very lucky little girl. I went back upstairs, found the place where she'd slipped into, and closed that sucker up for good! I didn't want either of us to go through that again. The final step was to fix the hole in the wall. It's amazing what sheetrock tape, some spackle, and a little paint can do. It looked almost as if nothing had happened. In the end, – we dodged a bullet, -no harm, no foul, – Willow wasn't injured, and some necessary corrections were made. The whole incident was pretty funny, – and just plain weird.

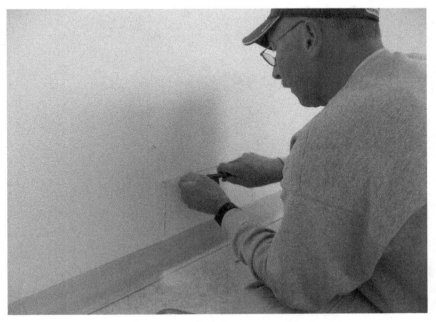

Doc operating on the wall to rescue "Willow"

Yikes

W e've all heard it, – that ubiquitous disclaimer statement heralded on the radio and television, – "Do not attempt this at home!". Most people pay attention and take note, – but some don't, – not good! Several disastrous "home-done" veterinary procedures come to mind, and validate the ole saying, "The road to hell is paved with good intentions".

Case number one involved a weekend "hobby" farmer named Dell and his one year old mixed breed male dog named, "Buddy". Dell's 15 acre retreat allowed him to have a small herd of cows that calved each year and he took care of all their medical needs himself, which is understandable. Unfortunately, treatments that work with one species of animals may not work very well when applied to another species. Dell learned this fact the hard way, and Buddy was the unlucky victim.

Dell brought Buddy to the veterinary clinic to be seen for a "licking problem". "Buddy is licking his rear end almost constantly." Dell said. "It looks infected. It stinks, and he won't leave it alone." Buddy was a good boy, – a little on the submissive side, as evidenced by his head lowered and having his tail slightly tucked between his hind legs. A few reassuring words, and a couple gentle pats on his head got him to relax somewhat before beginning the exam. The distinct, sickening odor of decaying flesh and the sight of saliva and serum soaked, matted hair in his groin area more than hinted that Buddy had a major problem going on. Moving Buddy's tail to the side exposed the gruesome details.

His scrotum was swollen and discolored, plus there were a few places where the skin looked necrotic, – grey-green, – dead, and was sloughing. "Dell", I said. "I've got to place Buddy under a general anesthetic so we can properly clean this mess up and treat it, without him experiencing any pain or discomfort. – Okay? Dell agreed, – signed the surgical release forms, and we were good to go.

When Buddy was sleeping comfortably, the cleanup process began. The entire groin area was thoroughly washed with surgical soap, then dried, and finally shaved. It didn't take but an instant to see the source of Buddy's problems. At the base of his scrotum, right next to the abdomen, was a small, hard rubber ring, – an "Elastrater Band", – a method used by some farmers and ranchers to castrate bull calves. A specifically designed device is used to place the rubber band over the scrotum and testicles. Once that rubber band is in place, it exerts major constrictive pressure on the skin and blood vessels, – essentially stopping all the blood flow to the scrotum and testicles, – eventually causing all of the effected tissue to die from lack of oxygen, wither and fall off. A hideous, cruel, and very inhumane procedure, – in MY opinion, and one technique that should NEVER be used on dogs!

All the infected and devitalized tissue had to be surgically removed, – specifically the entire scrotum, testicles, and adjacent skin. Once that was completed, reconstruction of what remained began. It took a while, but eventually everything came together nicely. Buddy was given an antibiotic injection, placed on some pain meds, – transferred to a warm recovery cage, and slowly woke up, – minus a few parts.

I had a little sit-down chat with Dell following the surgery, and he definitely got the message, – no more banding, – PERIOD! That was a sad case of good intentions gone terribly wrong, and hopefully would never happen again. In the end, Buddy healed well, no complications, – all the licking stopped, – a lesson was learned, – and life was good.

Next Case #2

Next case, – sometimes you just have to shake your head and wonder, – "What were they thinking?", or "How'd they come up with that?". One thing's for sure, – a day in the life of a veterinarian is anything but dull!

I overheard our receptionist telling a caller that we couldn't just dispense antibiotics, the animal had to be examined by the doctor first and then he'd dispense the appropriate medications if needed. After Angela hung up the phone, I asked her, "What was that call all about?" "Oh, – it was somebody new. –We've never seen any of their animals before. The lady and her husband are nurses, – their dog has an infection, she said, – and she wanted us to sell her some antibiotics. I told her that we couldn't do that, – the dog had to be examined first, before any medications could be dispensed. The lady was a little upset, but then told me she'd have to talk it over with her husband." "You handled that really well, Angela." I commented. "The ball's in their court now. We'll see what happens."

The people brought their dog to the clinic the next day to be checked over. Their defensive body language and curt responses to questions indicated that they weren't especially pleased with the situation. They did explain that the dog had somehow cut itself, and that they sewed the wound back together by themselves, – since they were nurses.

The wound was located on the lower left side of the dog's abdomen. It looked pretty grody and there was a foul odor of moist hair mixed with saliva and pus. When I gently separated some of the matted hair, the inflamed, infected wound, along with several stitches, suddenly appeared. "WOWEE!" I told the owners,

"We've got a pretty good infection going on here. Did you guys clean out the wound before suturing it?" "No, – not really" The lady responded. "We didn't think that we had to take as many precautions, – because he's just an animal, – not human." "Well," I said. "unfortunately, their skin and tissue responds and heals much the same way that ours does, and requires the same medical procedures and treatments to ensure proper healing. What we've got here is a badly contaminated and infected wound that wasn't properly cleaned and prepped before stitching closed. There's most likely a lot of dirt, hair and bacteria locked inside, – and that's what's causing the problem. What we've got to do is shave the area, open the wound, thoroughly clean, debride, and disinfect the tissue, then properly suture (stitch) everything back together. He'll need to be placed an systemic antibiotics for a couple weeks too." His owners weren't especially thrilled, to put it mildly, but they finally agreed that something had to be done, and reluctantly signed the surgical release forms. At that point, we were good to go.

We placed the 40 pound "Heinz-57" mixed breed dog, named "Sam", under a general anesthetic. He was a good patient, – went out like a light, and when he was nice and comfortable, we started prepping him for surgery. Shaving off the messy, matted hair quickly exposed a very angry looking wound whose edges were being held in close proximity by four stitches placed about an inch apart. Greenish-yellow pus mixed with tacky serum was escaping from between the sutures, and the smell was horrendous! The ole saying, "the odor was so bad it could gag a maggot!" certainly applied in this case! A little dab of Vicks Vapo Rub up the nose did the trick, and quenched the stench. When the stitches were snipped, the wound instantly spread open, and revealed the source of the contamination, – lots of crud. The wound had NOT been cleaned before it was sutured shut, – locking large amounts of hair, dirt, and bacteria inside there, – not good! I removed the contaminants, then thoroughly cleaned, flushed, debrided, medicated, and finally sutured the wound closed. Problem solved!

"Sam" was placed on systemic antibiotics for ten days, and healed up nicely. A lesson had been learned, and hopefully Sam wouldn't have to go through that experience again.

Next Case #3

Wire and a pair of pliers are really handy around the farm. Those two things have their place, and can provide temporary fixes for a multitude of problems, – but there's a definite limit to their usefulness!

"Clyde" was an 80 pound, Yellow Labrador Retriever, about a year old or so, and his owner wanted to have the dog's "credentials" checked. Clyde came sauntering into the clinic as if he owned the place, – greeted everyone as if they were his long-lost friends, and then checked out the dog treat display for any available freebees. He was a "kool" dog. That happy-go-lucky guy was right on time for his appointment, so he didn't have to wait very long before being guided into exam room #2.

We got Clyde onto the hydraulic "lift" table, – elevated it up, – and raised his left hind leg to check his, – "credentials". – "WOWZA!!" Clyde's scrotum was very swollen, – almost twice normal size, badly discolored, and the whole area appeared wet, most likely from a combination of serum discharge and Clyde's saliva from his incessant licking to relieve the discomfort. There was also a strong "infected" odor emanating from his groin region. I gloved up and began a more thorough examination of the problem area, and almost immediately noticed something that looked like a piece of metal imbedded in the skin at the base of Clyde's scrotum. "What the heck!" I muttered to myself. "This is crazy!" At first I was dumbfounded, – then I realized it was a piece of metal wire, – that had been purposely placed there, – twisted tightly, with the loose ends sniped off. UNBELIEVEABLE1 I quickly turned to the owner and asked him with a disgusted tone in my voice, "Did you do this?" There was a brief pause before the guy responded. Then, he said with remorse, "Yeah, – but I didn't think it'd turn out this way." I explained to him that the dog's scrotum and testicles were badly infected, and the only recourse was to surgically remove the entire scrotum, testicles, and adjacent devitalized skin and tissue. Then reconstruct what was left. After getting the owner's permission, off to surgery we went. It took a while, but eventually we got him cleaned up and put back together. – good as new, – but minus a few parts. Clyde went home the next day, – was on antibiotic meds for a couple weeks, – and healed up with hardly a scar.

It never ceased to amaze me how well Labrador Retrievers tolerated pain. The breed, generally speaking, seemed to have a higher pain threshold than most other breeds of dogs. They could,– as the saying goes, – "take a licking and keep on ticking". They really were very good, – and forgiving patients.

A Box of Chocolates

There's a simple little phrase that almost everyone can relate to in one way or another. Here it is, – "Life is like a box of chocolates, you never know what you're gonna get." Heck, – almost every day at the veterinary clinic was like a box of chocolates, in a lot of ways, because you never knew what kind of animal or medical case might be coming through the door next. But, – that's what made the days interesting, challenging, – and definitely not boring.

A Mysterious Wound

The first appointment on the books that day simply stated, – "dog with wound on side". When I read that, all kinds of scenarios and possibilities came to mind, – was it a traumatic injury like a dog fight wound or a barbed wire cut? Was it large, – small – superficial, – deep? Was there major or minor tissue damage? Was it actively bleeding or not? Did it just happen or was it an old wound? I was just getting myself mentally prepared for the case.

It wasn't long before the clinic door opened and a very smartly dressed lady came waltzing in with an Australian Shepherd mixed breed dog in tow. At first glance the 40 pound dog didn't appear seriously wounded, – but first impressions are often misleading and frequently inaccurate. The lady stated that her dog, "Sky", was outside, in the yard, and was barking up a storm. "Sky barks a lot." She said. "But this time she was barking louder and more aggressively than usual. So I went out to see what was going on out there. I didn't see anything, – but she could have been barking at a deer. We've got lots of deer, – they come into the yard, and Sky tries to chase them off. Could they have attacked her?" "That's always a possibility." I replied. "Let's get her on the exam table and check her over.

Sky's hair coat was medium length, and there was a large area on her left side, along her ribcage, where the hair appeared scruffy, somewhat matted and moist, with evidence of blood. As I parted the hair to get a closer look, Sky let out a shrill "yip!" and recoiled in obvious pain. I told Sky's owner that I needed to clip some hair away to get a better view of the problem area, and the lady agreed. Sky wasn't very keen about the procedure, but I removed enough hair to see that there was a gaping wound under all that matted hair. I told the owner, "Sky needs to be sedated so I can get in there and repair the wound without her feeling any pain ." The owner gave her consent, – and Sky was given a general anesthetic. When she was resting comfortably in "dream land", the procedure began.

I clipped away a large area of hair on Sky's left chest, over her ribs. There wasn't just one wound, – there were two, and the skin was severely damaged, – roughly torn, with major skin and subcutaneous tissue trauma. It appeared as if there was a downward thrust to that area by a blunt object of some kind, which resulted in severely tearing Sky's skin and tissue. The entry wound, high on her ribcage, appeared to be about three inches wide, and extended downward about six inches to where the skin was once again split open. "What could have caused that?" I asked myself. The wound showed all the signs of blunt-force trauma. The quick downward thrust of a deer's hoof could very possibly produce that kind of wound. A deer's hoof is pointed, about 3 inches in width, and deer defend themselves by striking with their legs and hooves. Unfortunately for Sky, that's what probably happened.

Now, – time to surgically repair and reconstruct the mess. First the area and wounds were shaved, cleaned, scrubbed, disinfected, and medicated. Next, – all the compromised and devitalized tissue was surgically removed . Then the disconnected and torn muscle, subcutaneous tissue and skin were reconstructed and reattached. A small penrose drain was placed at the lowest point of the wound and the final procedure consisted of suturing the skin closed. Hey, – it looked almost as good as new! Sky was hospitalized for 24 hours to monitor her recovery, and she did just fine.

Sky's owner suspected that Sky had an altercation with a deer, – and I told her that she was spot on to assume that. I also told the owner that deer are very adept at defending themselves by quick and forceful thrusts with their legs and pointed hooves. Unfortunately Sky got in the way and suffered the consequences.

In the end, – all's well that ends well, as they say, and hopefully Sky had learned a valuable lesson., – keep a safe distance between you and a determined deer.

"A Piglet With An Attitude"

Pigs can be funny! Sometimes their antics really crack me up. I recall a time when I was a financially strapped veterinary student, with a family, and very limited funds for entertainment. We'd go to the Animal Science pig barns, for FREE, and watch the little piglets scurry around their VERY patient moms. They ran around, chasing each other, – little ears flapping, a lot of squealing, grunting, then suddenly stopping to grab a nipple and some milk from mom, – quiet for a millisecond, – then do it all over again. Those were good times, – great memories. So, it's no wonder that I enjoy pigs, – especially the piglets.

It was one of those "crazy" days at the veterinary clinic, – nothing was routine, – but that's what made the profession fun and interesting. You didn't know what you'd have to deal with next. It really was like a box of chocolates.

Harvey Miller called and was quite concerned about one of his sows. He told Pam, Our receptionist, that the pig had been in labor for a long time, – had been straining a lot, but nothing was happening. "She's pretty tuckered out." He said. "And I think she needs some help." I got on the phone, got some additional information from Mr. Miller, then told him that I'd be out to his place within the hour. Oh joy! I was about to become a pig mid-wife. Sows usually don't have much trouble farrowing (birthing piglets), but when they do, – things can get pretty tricky, – real fast, – help is definitely needed.

When I arrived at the Miller farm, Harvey was standing over there by the barn, nervously shuffling his feet. He looked like an expectant father waiting in a maternity ward. I stopped the rig, got out and asked Mr. Miller, "Where is she?" "In here. – She's in the barn." Harvey replied. I followed his lead, and there she was, laying flat out on her side, on a clean bed of straw in the far corner of the barn. It was a nice, quiet, semi-secluded spot.

"She's a Landrace" Harvey said. "About three years old, – this is her third litter. – She's never had any problems before. – I guess there's a first time for everything, huh! She's been a good pig, – good sized litters,– been healthy, – no problems, – till now." As I was setting my bucket and stuff down, I noticed the sow having a half-hearted contraction. She was a typical Landrace, – white, long bodied, floppy ears, – about 350-400 pounds. I knew she was pretty tuckered out when I inserted the rectal thermometer, because the ole gal barely moved. Her temperature was in the normal range, 101.5 -102.5 degrees Fahrenheit. A good sign! No apparent systemic infections or toxicities. Now, – time to go in there and see what's going on.

I gloved up, washed and cleaned the area around the vulva, –
then put on my O.B. (obstetric) glove, – applied some lubricant, –
then proceeded to insert my hand and arm into the place where the
sun doesn't shine. It was a tight fit! The sow grunted and vocal-
ized a low groan as I slowly and gently went through the narrow
birth canal. It was a delicate procedure because the lining tissue
had become swollen and edematous. As my hand approached the
opening to the uterus, – I suddenly felt a tiny snout with the tips of
my finger, but there was no movement. My first thought was that
the piglet was dead. Then, – quick as a wink, – the little snout wiggled! "Hey Harvey, – We've got a live one in here! – Now, to get
him out of there." As I started to move my fingers over the piglet's
snout he quickly pulled his head back out of my reach. I had to
insert my hand and arm a little deeper, and once again touched the
snout. When I attempted to grasp the little guy's nose, – WHAM!!
– "OUCH", – ZOWEE!!! That little poop bit my finger! Harvey
instantly saw the pained expression on my face and heard my, not
so subtle expletives. 'What's wrong?" Harvey blurted out. "That
piglet bit me! – He sunk his "Needle Teeth" right into my finger!
Man, that hurts! That boy doesn't want to come out,. He likes it in
there." I then attempted to get a grip on his little snout so I could
pull him out, but he bit the snot out of me. Piglets are born with 4
pair of Milk Teeth, also called Wolf Teeth, or Needle Teeth. They
are very sharp and pointed, and can do a lot of damage to the sows
nipples and to other piglets. Those little monsters needed to be
clipped off right after birth.

I cleaned off my bloody finger, – put on a new O.B. glove and
went back in, – with a new strategy in mind. Now, – the moment
I felt that pesky piglets' snout, – I opened my hand, extended my
fingers over and around that little guy's head, so that his nose was
touching the center of the palm of my hand, I quickly hooked
my fingers behind his head and ears, – and, – "GOT HIM"!!!

I then gently pulled that piglet, with an attitude, out from his hidey-hole and into the light of a whole new world. He wasn't too thrilled about the whole ordeal. It didn't take long before he started squealing in protest, as he zeroed in on a nipple.

Once that little trouble maker was out of the way, the floodgates opened, – the sow started having normal, rhythmical contractions, and more little piglets came popping out of there. She had a total of 11 piglets, – all normal and healthy. Harvey and I clipped off all those nasty needle teeth, and that little "problem" piglet was first in line.

It was now time for me to go back to the clinic and nurse my own wounds, but I still enjoyed matching wits with a pesky little piglet, – with an attitude.

"Ticked Off"

Springtime is a wonderful time of the year. The snowy, cold, dreary days of winter give way to sun, warmth, and a resurgence of life all around. Birds sing, flowers bloom, spirits are lifted, – and the dreadful ticks come out of hiding.

"Doc, there's a person on the phone who says her dog isn't walking right, and wonders if it should be seen." "Tell her to bring the dog right in!" I said. "There are a lot of things that can cause that, and some are pretty serious. So, – we need to examine it right now."

About 15 minutes later the clinic door opened and in came a lady with her dog that was walking and acting like a happy drunk. The 30 pound Spaniel-mix, named "Lucy", was excited and happy on the front end, but very weak and wobbly in the hindquarters. The dog seemed to be oblivious to the fact that her back end wasn't in sync with the front end, and there were no overt signs of pain. "Let's get Lucy on the exam table and check her over. I think I know what's going on here."

"What do you think it is, doctor?" The owner asked. – "Lucy is showing all the classic signs of Tick Paralysis." I replied. "Embedded ticks can secrete neurotoxins that interfere with nerve transmissions, – shuts them down, and then the muscles stop working properly. There's no feeling. It starts in the hindquarters and moves forward. The muscles become weak, – there's a loss of balance, the animal looks uncoordinated, and has difficulty walking. What we need to do is look for a tick and remove it immediately, so we can stop the neurotoxins from getting into Lucy's body. That's critical, because the paralysis continues to move forward. It's essentially a progressive anterior (forward) paralysis, and if it isn't stopped, – well, Lucy could be in serious trouble, – even die in a day or two if the tick isn't removed. The good thing though, is that when the tick is removed, no more neurotoxins get absorbed, and recovery can take place pretty fast. Sometimes, improvement can be seen in minutes or hours,. It all depends upon how much of the neurotoxin is in their system.

Everybody got into the act, – staff members, myself, and the owner. Lucy was totally "Lovin" it. She thought she was getting the "Royal Petting" treatment. Suddenly, one of the vet techs chimed out, "FOUND ONE!' I need a "tick puller"." (A Tick Puller is a little device that can remove the entire tick along with the embedded head of the tick.) I told the owner that if she didn't have a Tick Puller, then a tweezer can also be used to gently pull the tick out, but NEVER, NEVER burn the tick with a hot object or match, and don't attempt to suffocate the tick with creams, ointments or anything like that. That would only stress the tick and cause it to regurgitate more neurotoxins into the animal. We continued searching, – found another tick, – and removed that dude too!

Lucy was having a great time, – and thoroughly enjoyed the whole experience. She thought that she'd come to the clinic for a big game of "Scratch & Tickle", but believe me, – it was a lot more serious than that. Actually, it was a matter of life or death!

We kept Lucy at the veterinary clinic for observation for a couple hours, and it was remarkable how rapidly the paralysis resolved. Lucy regained her muscle strength and showed improved coordination in her hindquarters within an hour and was almost back to normal two hours later. It was, – simply AMAZING!

Lucy's owner pledged to become more proactive about tick prevention and to be more diligent about looking for and removing ticks from her other animals. This was just another "Box of Chocolates" case.

"What Just Happened?"

Life is full of surprises. Unexpected things can, and do, happen, – to all of us. There was one particular "surprising" case at the veterinary clinic that comes to mind. What was supposed to be a simple, routine exam turned out to be something very different.

A new client recently purchased a three month old Bassett puppy and scheduled an appointment to have his new little friend checked over and vaccinated. Puppy exams are most always fun, and the entire staff was looking forward to this one because Bassett puppies are so dang cute, especially with those big sad eyes and extra long ears.

When the new client entered the clinic, he didn't appear to be carrying a puppy, but his arms were gently cradling an oversized lump in the front of his jacket. Suddenly, without warning, a little tri-colored head with very long ears, popped out above the zipper. That not so subtle move, instantly precipitated a chorus of "Oohs and Ahs" from everyone who witnessed it.

The owner and his new best buddy named, "Barney", were ushered into exam room #1. Barney was definitely a "chick magnet" and all the adoring attention got him pretty hyped-up and excited. So, in an attempt to calm the little guy down a bit, one of the vet techs placed a bowl of puppy food in front of him. Barney dove into that bowl like he'd never seen food before. Suddenly, without warning, Barney did a perfect "face plant" directly into the center of the bowl of food, – scattering kibbles all over the place!

Barney just laid there, – limp, –motionless. I quickly checked his mouth and throat to make sure that he wasn't choking, then grabbed the stethoscope, – listened to his heart and lungs, – his heart was beating normally, – respirations were regular and deep, – his mucous membrane color was nice and pink. Barney was basically, – ASLEEP! Then, without any fanfare, – Barney suddenly WOKE UP, – looked around at everybody, wagged his tail, and promptly returned to eating his kibbles.

"What just happened?" Barney's owner exclaimed, – half in shock himself. "Did he have a heart attack, a seizure, or something? That was just weird!" "Yeah, it was." I replied. It sure looks like a condition called narcolepsy, or it could be cataplexy." "What the heck is that?" The owner asked. "It's a disorder in the nervous system." I responded. And it's seen primarily in the young animals. It's not very common, – actually pretty rare. It doesn't seem to be painful, they usually don't get hurt, and it's not a fatal condition either. Barney is the first case of narcolepsy I've ever seen, and I think I'm spot on because he's showing all the classic signs of the condition.

A narcoleptic episode involves sudden collapse and unconsciousness. The animal really does, – literally, fall asleep, – then abruptly wakes up, and acts like nothing has happened. The episodes only last for a brief period of time, – a few seconds to minutes in most cases, but to any bystander it seems like hours." "What causes these things, Doc?" The owner asked. "Well," I said. "Most seem to be brought on by periods of excitement, – like playing or eating, and that's especially true with cataplexy. So in Barney's case, less is more as far as excitement goes. He'll need quieter eating times, and controlled play and activity time where he doesn't get too wound up. The good news is, – they usually outgrow the condition in the great majority of cases. The odds are good that Barney won't have any more of these episodes once he gets a little older. Barney's owner understood and was much relieved. Barney, on the other hand, was oblivious to the whole thing, and just wanted more pets and goodies. Uh, – be careful!!!

Barney's first visit to our veterinary clinic was one that I'll never forget, and neither will anyone else who was there and witnessed the spectacle. Barney's narcolepsy – cataplexy episode was a definite surprise, but surprises are just a fact of life. Some are enjoyable, – others, not so much. – The ole "Box of Chocolates" thing again.

Unconditional Love

U nconditional love is often defined as affection without limi-
tations, to love someone as they are, — completely, — without reservation, — and in all circumstances. That close, unselfish
relationship can often exist between animals and their human
companions, and in many cases, both have their lives enriched
and prolonged by the experience.

"Juliette"

Strays tend to be independent creatures who are, "On the lam".
They've either run away from a bad situation, been abandoned, or
have simply remained feral. Strays essentially are out there operating in survival mode, — focusing on two basic needs, — food
and shelter. When they find a place where food is plentiful and the
shelter is safe and secure, they seize the moment, and often hang
up their nomadic lifestyle, — and settle in. In many instances,
if given a chance, these vagabonds can often become wonderful
friends and faithful companions.

A four year old domestic shorthair cat of unknown ancestry
was out there on her own, — a stray. I don't exactly know how
Kim Olson crossed paths with the unkept feline, but she felt sorry
for the little waif. Kim thought the cat had probably been abandoned, and decided to befriend the poor little thing and take her
home. The cat quickly adjusted to her new surroundings and Kim
soon came to the realization that another cat had been added to the
household. She figured that if the cat was going to stay, it needed

a proper name, so Kim named the little ragamuffin, "Juliette". It wasn't long before a strong bond of love and trust was forged between the two of them, and it continued to mature through the years.

Juliette was about nine years old when when she came to the clinic for her annual checkup and vaccinations. She appeared to be healthy and happy, but while examining her mouth, I noticed a small, hard, bean-sized lump on the right side of her lower jaw, near her mandibular canine tooth. I asked Kim, "How long has Juliette had this lump on her jaw?" Kim replied, "Not too long, — I guess. I thought it might be an infected tooth or something, — maybe a little abscess, because she does get into some fisticuffs with the other cats once in a while." As I continued to examine the lump, I found it to be very firm, non-movable, it wasn't painful or warm to the touch, and the adjacent lymph nodes weren't enlarged, — yet. "What do you think's going on, Doc?" Kim asked, with some definite concern in her voice. "It could be an infected tooth, an encapsulated abscess, a bone infection, or a bone tumor." I replied. "Most infections tend to be uncomfortable and the animals usually have elevated temps, but Juliette's temp is normal, and the lump doesn't seem to be that painful to her when I press on it." — I hesitated a few moments before continuing, then I told her, "Kim, — I seriously believe that we're looking at a tumor here, — bone cancer, — an osteosarcoma, — and that kind of tumor isn't very forgiving. — they're usually malignant. An x-ray should tell us if that's what's going on here." Tears began to well up in Kim's eyes as she said, "Oh Juliette, why'd this have to happen to you?" X-rays were taken and showed significant bone changes that were consistent with bone cancer, — and the prognosis wasn't good. When Kim asked how long Juliette had, I told her that Juliette had perhaps six to nine months, maybe a year to live. My heart felt heavy as I spoke those words, — it was always difficult delivering bad news. Radiation treatments and chemotherapy were options, and could possibly give Juliette some additional time, — but there were no guarantees. Kim realized that, and decided not to subject Juliette to all the treatments. She just wanted Juliette to be comfortable for as long as possible. Quality of life was Kim's primary concern. I completely understood and wholeheartedly agreed with her decision. I told Kim that I'd taken that approach with my own animals when they had cancers, and I'd be willing to treat Juliette as if she were my very own. Kim smiled wistfully and nodded her head in approval. She needed a hug, — so I gave her a consoling embrace. I knew how she felt, — I'd been there myself.

I placed Juliette on pain medication and anti-inflammatory drugs in an effort to make her more comfortable, and slow the rate of tumor growth. I checked her frequently over the ensuing six months, and as the tumor grew, so did the degree of disfigurement of Juliette's face, but the love connection between Kim and Juliette never faltered. Their relationship was the perfect example of mutual unconditional love and devotion.

It had been almost ten months since Juliette was first diagnosed with bone cancer, and the time had now come to help her gently cross over to the other side. Kim and Juliette had supported each other through some very tough times, yet their mutual affection never wavered. That committed resolve enabled them to endure till the end.

"Abigail"

Abigail was a Siamese-cross cat whose better years were behind her. When she was twelve years old, her owner, Mary Mills, noticed that Abigail was getting thinner, in spite of her voracious appetite. Abigail was still her happy, active self, but the progressive weight loss concerned Mary, so she made an appointment to have Abigail examined.

Mary entered the exam room, clutching a very thin cat in her arms. The cat seemed perfectly content as it periodically gazed up at Mary. My physical exam of Abigail revealed an active, older cat, who looked like a starvation case, — basically skin and bones. Although her eyes were bright and lungs sounded clear, her heart beat was quite loud and rapid. When I offered her a few cat treats, she devoured them without chewing, and then frantically looked for more. I told Mary there were many factors that could contribute to a cat losing weight so rapidly. The most likely were malabsorption syndrome, parasites, diabetes, hyperthyroidism, and cancer. Several diagnostic tests needed to be performed in order to narrow the field of possibilities. The fecal analysis was negative, so internal parasites were not an issue. Abigail's lymph nodes were not enlarged, she didn't have any visible tumors, and most cancer cases weren't as active and animated as she was. Her blood analysis showed normal blood glucose levels, so she didn't appear to be diabetic, and she wasn't anemic or leukemic. However, the results of the T4 test, a blood test used to evaluate the thyroid activity, was extremely elevated!!!! Abigail had a hyperthyroid condition, — her metabolism was working at warp speed, — burning up all her fat reserves. That's why she was losing weight, even though she was eating voraciously. Her body was running on "high idle", which contributed to the rapid heart rate. The poor little cat may have appeared calm on the outside while resting in Mary's arms, but she had a raging metabolism on the inside. That's why she looked so thin, — as if she was starving, — she couldn't eat enough to maintain a normal body weight.

I told Mary that there were several treatment options for hyperthyroid conditions,—surgical removal of the thyroid gland, radiation therapy to destroy the gland, or oral medication to slow down the thyroid gland's activity. Mary selected the oral medication. Abigail was a very good patient, and I checked her T4 values periodically to make medication dosage adjustments if necessary. Mary faithfully gave Abigail the medication, and demonstrated that beauty really was in the eye of the beholder. Mary was totally committed to loving and caring for Abigail, no matter what the situation or circumstance. That display of unconditional love and devotion allowed little Abigail to gain some weight and live comfortably for nineteen years.

"Shelby"

Barbara Wilson was one of the most compassionate, empathetic individuals that I'd ever met. Her snow white hair, radiant smile, positive attitude about life, and genuine love for animals and their welfare, definitely set her apart. It was always a joy to see her walk through that clinic door.

Barbara had recently adopted a dog from the local humane society and it was scheduled for a courtesy health check and physical exam. I shouldn't have been surprised by her selection, but I was. You see, the dog wasn't exactly what most people would have chosen to rescue, but once again, Barbara wasn't like most people. The dog was a middle-aged spayed female Brittany Spaniel -Shelty cross with a right ear that permanently stuck out to the side as if signaling to make a turn, and weak facial muscles on the right side of her head which suggested some previous traumatic nerve injury or side effects from a stroke. Her hair coat wasn't that great either. It appeared dull and brittle, something often seen as a result of poor nutrition. Curiosity got the best of me, so I asked Barbara, "Why'd you choose this dog?" "I liked her, — and she's a nice girl." Barbara glanced wistfully at the dog and responded, "Nobody seemed to want her, and I felt sorry for the poor little thing, — so I thought I'd give her a chance,

— she deserved at least that much. Everybody deserves a chance, —don't you think?" I nodded my head in agreement, continued the exam, and proceeded to point out some of the dog's physical flaws. Barbara looked down at the dog, smiled, and reassuringly said, — "I know." That was good enough for me, so I told her that I'd do all I could to help the little girl.

Barbara had named the dog, "Shelby", but in my opinion, it should have been named "Blessed", because it was truly blessed to have been adopted by such a loving and caring person. The first order of business was to get Shelby on some quality food, and it didn't take long before her hair coat was shiny and supple. She still had flaccid facial muscles and a droopy upper eyelid on her right side, but she was happy and very devoted to Barbara. Those two sure loved each other.

Several years passed by, and on one of Shelby's routine annual exams, I noticed that the hair on her torso and hind legs was thinning. She also didn't seem as energetic and animated as before, in fact, she appeared quite lethargic. I told Barbara that I needed to draw some blood and test Shelby's thyroid activity. The test results revealed that her T4 value was definitely BELOW normal, Shelby was hypothyroid, the the thyroid gland was not functioning as it should, and that contributed to her hair loss and sluggishness. I immediately placed her on medication to specifically stimulate the thyroid gland. Barbara conscientiously gave Shelby the meds as directed. Shelby's hair grew back nicely, she wasn't lethargic anymore, and she quickly returned to her normal, active self. Problem solved, — but she needed to stay on the medication and have her thyroid values checked every few months for any dosage adjustments.

All went well for two more years, but then Shelby started showing different signs that raised some concerns. She was drinking more water and consequently urinating more. Her skin, especially on the abdomen, appeared thinner and more wrinkled than normal, and she had muscle weakness, especially in the hind legs. These findings raised a red flag for Cushing's disease, a disease that involves the adrenal gland. A routine blood chemistry screen showed that her serum alkaline phosphatase was elevated, as well as the serum cholesterol levels, and the leukogram (white blood cell analysis) revealed some signs of stress. I then ran a high-dose dexamethasone suppression test and a urine cortisol:creatine ratio test, and the results of both tests confirmed my suspicions. Shelby now had Cushing's disease syndrome along with her hypothyroid condition, and she needed to be placed on medication to shrink down the adrenal gland and slow its activity. There was, however, one major problem. The medication of choice made Shelby very sick. She vomited, had diarrhea, and refused to eat. NOT GOOD! There were other methods of treatment available, including surgical removal of the adrenal gland and radiation therapy, but Barbara wasn't interested. My options were getting smaller, pretty fast. I recalled reading an article in a resent veterinary journal about a new drug being used in England to treat Cushing's disease in dogs, and it was reported to be very safe and effective. BINGO! That would be just the ticket for Shelby. — I had to get ahold of some of that stuff. Then came the "fly in the ointment". —The drug wasn't yet available in the United States for veterinary use, — but I did manage to find out that there was a company in Boston that could import the medication through Canada. I phoned the company, and ordered a bottle right then and there. Barbara was excited about the new find, and with her permission, Shelby was started on the new drug. It worked great! She had no side effects, and in short order the little dog with the sticky-outy ear and weak facial muscles was enjoying life again.

Everyone has heard the saying, "things happen in threes", and in Shelby's case it unfortunately was true. The following year, during a routine physical exam, I detected a heart murmur, and some lung congestion, which explained why she'd recently been coughing more than usual. X-rays showed that the poor little girl's heart was enlarged because the muscles had become stretched and weakened as a result of the tricuspid mitral valve not closing properly, — which produced the murmur. The heart valve problem was not allowing the left side of the heart to efficiently pump the oxygenated blood from the lungs out throughout her body. As a result, there was back pressure into the lungs, and this caused fluid to accumulate in the lungs (pulmonary edema), and the reason for the cough. I placed Shelby on vasodilator medication for the heart and diuretics to remove fluid from the lungs. Her diet was also changed to a special cardiac diet which was low in sodium (salt), so as to decrease fluid retention. Shelby responded well to the treatment, the cough stopped, and the heart problem was managed successfully from that time forward.

Barbara Wilson and Shelby epitomized an unconditional love relationship, and it greatly enriched both of their lives. Barbara really loved that unusual looking little dog, she gave it a chance just like she said it deserved, and faithfully cared for it through all its health challenges. Shelby and Barbara were a blessing to each other, and their close, unselfish relationship got them through the tough times, and allowed them to have many wonderful years together.

Catch of the Day

Living and working in a small town surrounded by five very productive fishing lakes was absolutely wonderful! Heck, there were many times when I'd go fishing at five o'clock in the morning, catch my limit of rainbow trout, clean them, and be at the veterinary clinic at eight A.M. to see my first patient of the day. It was really a kick in the pants, and I wasn't the only one who enjoyed the fishing either. The lakes were like magnets, drawing people from miles around with their boats, dogs, fishing poles and tackle boxes full of fishing gear. Everyone seemed to be having a good time, — until something went wrong, — and when trouble hit, — it usually involved a fishhook.

Those brightly colored, flashy fishing lures dangling on the end of a line or flying through the air were too tempting for most dogs. They'd instinctively leap and and snap at the "flying toy", and many, unfortunately, suffered the consequences. Some people got real creative and even put a smorgasbord of marshmallows, tasty red worms, and yellow stinky bait around the hook. That tantalizing morsel proved too much for some dogs, — and down the hatch it went. — Time to go to the vet!

Most of the time the barbed hooks got painfully embedded in the dog's lip, and the angled barb prevented the hook from being pulled out. The only solution was to sedate the dog, and then painlessly push the tip of the hook completely through the lip. Once that was accomplished and the barb was exposed, a side-cutter tool was then used to cut off and remove the barbed end. Now, the remainder of the hook could be easily removed. It was a whole different story, however, when a dog swallowed the smorgasbord.

Everything had been quite routine that day at the clinic until an unannounced emergency came through the front door. "My dog just swallowed a fishhook, and I think it's really down there." The owner said. His forty pound "Heinz-57" dog just stood there, flipping its tongue at the monofilament fishing line hanging out of its mouth. I quickly sedated the dog, whose name was Rufus, and took x-rays to identify the type of hook and pinpoint its location. The x-rays revealed that the dog had swallowed a triple hook, and it was located at the bottom end of the esophagus, right next to the entry opening into the stomach. The owner was right, — it was way down there! Now the big question, — how to get it out of there! The triple hook couldn't simply be pulled out because all three hooks would then sink deeply into the esophageal tissue. Attempting to move and reposition the hook directly into the stomach, and then retrieving it via abdominal surgery and a gastrotomy was a possible option, but much more complicated and time consuming. I didn't own a gastroscope to maneuver down the esophagus to grasp the hook, but a nearby veterinary specialist did, — unfortunately their office was closed. As I was mulling over my options, — I suddenly had an epiphany! I recalled a seldom used instrument that I'd purchased several years earlier, and the thought occurred to me that it might be helpful in this particular case. The special instrument was a tubular scope about 18 inches long and 1/2 inch in diameter, with a built in light source. I muttered to myself, — "This might actually work!"

I began the procedure by threading the monofilament fishing line through the tube. Thank goodness the owner didn't cut the line any shorter than he did. I then carefully moved the scope down the esophagus while maintaining light tension on the line until the shiny triple hook came into view. I gently dislodged the hook with the tip of the scope, and managed to snag one of the hooks on the rim of the scope. Then, while maintaining light traction on the line, I carefully withdrew the scope along with the hook from the confines of the esophagus. YAHOO! It worked!

Rufus did great! He recovered quickly and didn't have any complications. I guess you could say that he was the "catch and release" patient of the day. Hopefully everyone, especially the dog, learned a lesson from the whole painful experience.

Reflections

W e've all experienced special moments in our lives that have produced lasting memories, — most of which were good, thank heavens. Some memories can fade over time, while others continue to endure. The following are a few amusing snippets from my memory bank.

"Lobo"

Lobo was a German Shepherd who honorably served in Viet Nam as a guard dog. Upon completion of his tour of duty, he somehow managed to defy the odds and made it back to the United States. This was, in all honesty, a minor miracle, because most dogs never left country. He eventually ended up living the remainder of his years on a small ranch located only a few miles from the clinic.

One might think that this dog's military training and wartime experiences would render him to be potentially dangerous and unacceptable for adoption, but that wasn't the case at all. The loud and threatening sounds of war were long gone. Lobo seemed to know that his military days were over, and it was now time for some well deserved R&R. He was a good boy, and his laid back personality was not unlike that of Ferdinand the bull. Instead of sitting amongst the flowers in a pasture, Lobo spent much of his time lounging in the sun with his adoring horde of cats. It was a mutual love affair between that dog and his feline companions.

The image of Lobo that will be forever etched in my memory occurred when I went on a farm call to the ranch to work on one of the horses. When I got out of the truck, there was Lobo, sauntering across the farmyard, surrounded by eight cats with "happy tails" lifted high in the air. He looked like some sort of rock star with his groupies.

Lobo was a great dog who lived life to the fullest, and actually made it to the ripe old age of nineteen, a feat most German Shepherds aren't fortunate enough to attain.

"Lobo"

"Cy"

It was one of those beautiful Spring Saturdays when everything was going right. The trees were leafed out, the lawn looked lush and green, and the flowers were beginning to bloom. Then suddenly, my moment in nirvana was interrupted by a stray cat jetting through my backyard as if he were trying to evade the IRS. His low profile running posture made it look like he was trying to avoid a barrage of low flying bullets. This guy was running scared.

It took some doing, but I managed to find the brown tabby cat hunkered down by the woodpile. He was young, about two to three years old, and I noticed there was something unusual about his appearance. Upon closer inspection, his eyes seemed to be positioned closer together than most cats. I squatted down and gently said to him, "Hey there little buddy, — I'm not going to hurt you. — What's your name?" The cat shifted his eyes and blinked several times. Then out came a high pitched —— Meowph! I continued talking to the little guy while slowly getting closer to him. He started to relax a little, feeling less threatened, and that's when the lispy meowing really started in earnest. — Meowph, — Meow-ph, — Meow-ph. I finally managed to get close enough to stroke his head, and that's when he actually started to purr. This frightened and homeless little cat was all alone in unfamiliar surroundings because he'd probably been dropped off and abandoned.

It didn't take long to gain his trust and confidence, and that enabled me to get close enough to pick him up and hold his trembling body in my reassuring arms. Now, the next hurdle, — find this little cat with the close set eyes and the lispy meow a good home. I took the little fella to the clinic for a thorough physical exam, deworming, vaccinations, and blood tests for feline leukemia and feline AIDS. He passed with flying colors, — but he needed an identity, — a name. Since his eyes were positioned so close together, — I decided to name him, "Cy", — short for cyclops.

Cy quickly settled into his new digs. He was a real charmer, and easily won over the hearts of the entire staff. Heidi, one of our veterinary technicians was smitten with him, and needless to say, Cy couldn't have found a better home. He was one of my favorite rescue cases. Cy was definitely one of a kind, — the cat with close set eyes was and a lisp, —— Meow-ph!

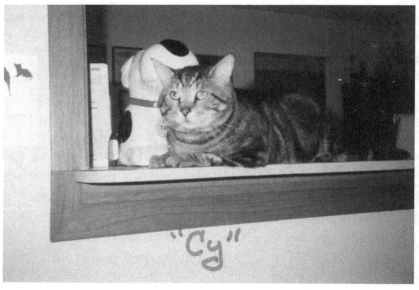

"Cy"

"Kindle"

A smiling dog is one thing that's sure to make almost anyone laugh. Those light-hearted canine expressions ranged from the wistful Mona Lisa type smiles to the big toothy grins that looked very much like a threatening snarl. Sometimes those funny facial expressions were accompanied by gentle whines, squinted or winking eyes, and even gyrating hindquarters. It was really a hoot! Over the years I saw quite a few smiling dogs, but there was one special little Pomeranian named, "Kindle", — and she was one smiler which I'll never forget.

Harvey Kranek called the clinic and inquired about purchasing a dog shampoo that would treat dry skin and dandruff. He'd recently bought a dog in Montana and it had been itching and scratching ever since he brought the dog home. He called the breeder and was told that the puppy just had dry, flaky skin, and that a little extra oil in the food and a good bath should solve the problem. The oil added to the food and a basic dog shampoo didn't seem to help, so Harvey was looking for a "stronger" shampoo. Our receptionist told Mr. Kranek that many things could contribute to a dog itching, and highly recommended that the dog be examined. Mr. Kranek was at his wits' end, and knew that something had to be done for the poor little dog, so he scheduled an appointment.

Several days later Mr. Kranek walked into the exam room, clutching a six month old tan-orange colored Pomeranian puppy named "Kindle". She was a cute little thing and I could definitely see why the Kranek family chose her. When you'd say her name and gently pat her on the head, she'd squint her little eyes and slightly draw up the corners of her mouth. I commented to Mr. Kranek, "Have you noticed that she smiles when she's happy?" Harvey responded, "Yeah. I know. Isn't that the funniest thing you've ever seen?" We both had a good chuckle. It actually seemed like the more we laughed, the more she smiled. It was crazy!

Now, down to business. Kindle could hardly stand still. She'd scratch almost nonstop at her back and sides with her hind paw. She was one very miserable little girl. I continued with the physical exam, and didn't see any fleas or flea dirt (droppings consisting of dried blood), — but there was flakey dandruff everywhere. I told Harvey that Kindle could have a mite infestation, and I needed to examine some of her hair and dandruff under the microscope. I took samples, placed them on a slide, focused in the microscope, and — BONANZA! We'd struck the mother lode! There, right before my eyes, were three chubby little Cheyletiella mites with their four sets of stubby legs moving in ultra slow motion. A few Cheyletiella eggs were lazily floating around on the slide too. I asked Harvey if he'd like to take a look. He was game. "There's the culprit." I said. "That's why Kindle is itching and scratching so much, and why she has all that dandruff." I told Harvey that Cheyletiella mite cases are often referred to as "walking dandruff" because the mites make the dandruff move ever so slightly. He thought that little fact was pretty neat, — but I was sure that Kindle wasn't amused. She was too focused on scratching.

There were several treatment options available. Some were systemic (absorbed by the body), and some were non-systemic. Since Kindle was young and weighed only 3 1/2 pounds, I felt the systemic treatments could possibly pose a safety risk. So, I selected a non-systemic therapeutic shampoo which contained pyrethrins, a safer insecticide compound. Harvey was instructed to bathe Kindle weekly for four weeks and wash all her bedding weekly as well. I was confident that treatment regimen would work, — and it did! Kindle got relief with the very first therapeutic bath, but Harvey followed through and completed the course of bathing as directed, and when the treatment was finished, Kindle looked and acted like a new dog. Her hair coat was soft and shiny, the dandruff was totally gone, and best of all, — she didn't itch anymore. One thing didn't change though, — she still smiled. I fondly recall each time Kindle visited the clinic. I'd say, "Hey Kindle, how's my girl?" She'd shyly dip her head slightly, squint those little brown eyes, and "smile". Kindle was a delight, and without a doubt, one of my sweetest patients.

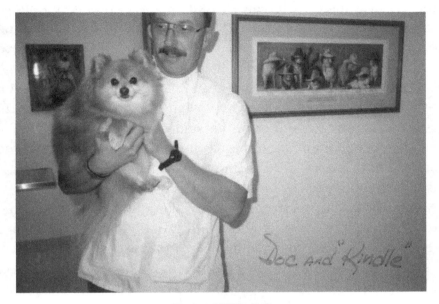

Doc and "Kindle"

Ask, And You Shall Receive

A farm call to the Neuland ranch was like taking a trip to Comedy Central — on the farm. The two hard working ranch hands, Skip and Bill, found humor in just about everything, and it was always a blast working with those two guys. Actually, it was more like having Cheech and Chong as assistants.

The ranch's cattle herd was on a routine deworming program, and periodic fecal exams were needed to evaluate the effectiveness of the medication. I'll never forget the time I called the ranch and asked Skip to drop off a small stool sample from the cows. Several days later a personally addressed letter to, "Doc Roloff", arrived in the mail. When I opened the envelope, I found a piece of facial tissue with a skid mark of cow manure on it. A small hand written note was also enclosed. It read, "Doc, here's the small sample you wanted." Signed, — Skip. I got a good laugh out of it, and so did everyone else in the clinic, — but I needed a tad more manure in order to run the test. So I called Skip, and when he recognized that it was me on the phone, he about "split-a-gut" laughing. "Doc", he said. "You got the letter, huh? You said you wanted a little sample, — so that's what we sent ya." Then there was more howling laughter on his end of the phone. He gave a tongue-in-cheek apology, in between snickers, and then told me that he'd drop off a "good" sample at the clinic in a few days. I fell for that one too.

Skip was true to his word. Two days later Skip and Bill walked through the clinic door, laughing and proudly carrying a frisbee piled high with fresh cow manure. My mind instantly conjured up all kinds of images of how they got that much poop on the frisbee, but the sample was sufficient. It was a weirdly comedic scene, — two guffawing sunshine boys, dressed in coveralls, holding a frisbee filled to overflowing, with aromatic cow dung. As I took the frisbee and its contents, I asked the guys if they wanted the frisbee back. They commented, "Nah. — You can keep it." Then more howling laughter. —— They got me again. Oh, by the way, the stool specimen was negative for parasite eggs, and if any additional tests would have been needed, —believe me, — there was more than enough dung available.

House Calls

House calls provided me the opportunity to witness firsthand, the positive interaction between people and their pets, — on their turf, instead of mine. It was always amazing to see how strong the human-animal bond could be, and observe the close relationship that often exists between soul mates.

Little Orphan Annie

As I walked into the clinic that morning, I couldn't help noticing a new patient in one of the recovery room cages. It was a noisy little tortoise-shell colored kitten, about six-teen weeks old, and she was very insistent about getting some attention. The cage card simply read, "Stray". I couldn't resist that cute little poop, so I opened the cage door and she instantly jumped into my arms and started purring. I looked down at her contented little face and asked her, "Sweetheart, who the heck are you, — and what's a nice girl like you doing in a place like this?" She didn't say much, but it was evident that she was overjoyed to get out of that cage and just be held.

It wasn't long before I got filled in on all the details. Melody, one of our veterinary assistants, had a neighbor suddenly move out of their rented home. They either knowingly or unknowingly left behind a very pregnant cat to fend for herself. The poor little mother-to-be was scared stiff, and sought refuge under the vacated house. She went from having food constantly available to frantic scavenging for anything that was edible, — but she was a true survivor. Melody set out food and water for the little abandoned waif, and that in itself was a life-saver. Soon the cat delivered four beautiful kittens, and Melody spent many hours socializing the kittens with hopes of finding them good homes. In time, three of the kittens had been placed, and Melody brought the remaining kitten, who she'd named "Annie", to the clinic for routine vaccinations, deworming, and possible adoption.

When Melody mentioned adoption, one person instantly came to mind, — Collin Sumpter. Collin was a bachelor who loved his cats, and he'd recently lost his beloved cat, "Callo". He was heartbroken, and told me that since Callo had been such a huge part of his life, it would probably take a long time before he'd be able to have another cat. I completely understood, because the grieving process can often take a while, but then Annie came on the scene two weeks later. I remembered what Mr. Sumpter had said, but I thought I'd give him a phone call anyway, and try to convince him to at least take a look at Annie. When Mr. Sumpter answered the phone, there was profound sadness in his voice. He wasn't at all receptive to the idea of getting another cat, so soon after Callo's passing. Perhaps he was patronizing me, but eventually he said, "I'll stop by sometime." Our conversation didn't leave me very optimistic, but it must have moved Mr. Sumpter, because later that day he came to the clinic and asked to see the kitten. When I walked into the exam room with Annie in my arms, Mr. Sumpter's face lit up like a neon sign and he smiled ear-to-ear as I handed him the kitten. Collin gently and lovingly stroked the kitten as he held it close to his chest. "What's its name?" He asked. "Annie, —— Little Orphan Annie." I said. He was totally smitten with that little cat, who was now thoroughly engrossed with Mr. Sumpter and all the attention he was giving to her. Then he said with a smile, "Little Orphan Annie, huh? —— I like that name. —— Would you like to come home with me?" I'd become a mere bystander, —— witnessing two needy individuals finding a soul mate in each other. It couldn't have worked out any better. —— They really looked like a match made in heaven.

Those two became devoted companions, and Mr. Sumpter provided Annie with the best of everything. Nothing was too good for his Annie. When it came time to go to the vet for her annual check-up and vaccinations, Collin requested that I make a house call, because he thought that would be less stressful for Annie. I agreed, and set up a time.

House calls were fun, —— most of the time. Invariably, the cat would disappear the moment I stepped inside the door. The most common owner comment was, "Where'd she go? She was here just a minute ago." The usual hiding places were either under the bed, behind the big chair, or under the couch. It often turned into a hands and knees exercise, with the coffee table or dinette doubling as an exam table, but it all seemed to work out just fine! Annie, although a quiet protester, was still a very good patient. She had her favorite escape routes and "safe" places. Hiding under Collin's bed seemed to be the default location, and that was the first place we looked. It was quite the scene, —— three people on their hands and knees, —— butts in the air, —— looking under the bed. All the while, trying to entice Annie from her safe haven with words of sweet nothings. Eventually the job got done, and we all had a good chuckle over what we put ourselves through for our feline friends.

Annie was the apple of Collin Sumpter's eye. His face would light up when he'd share stories of Annie's antics and perceptive abilities. He was also emphatic about the fact that cats can teach us alot about life, —— if only we'd take the time to know them as true friends and devoted companions.

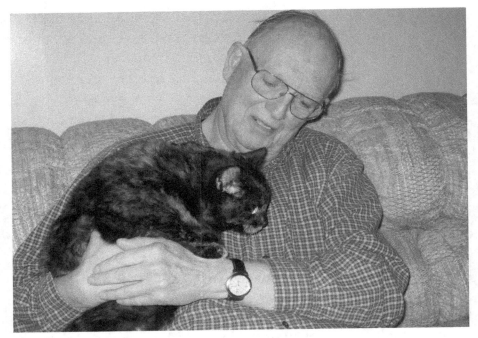

"Little Orphan Annie" with Collin

One of a Kind

Mr. Konig was a spry little gent in his eighties who had a soft spot in his heart for cats. He was our local, "Saint Francis" of cats on Lake and LeFevre streets, befriending any sick and abandoned felines, and bringing them to our veterinary clinic for care and treatment. Thank heavens for the generous donations to our "compassion fund", because those funds helped defray some of the medical costs incurred with treating all those strays.

As time passed, it was becoming increasingly more difficult for Mr. Konig to catch his own cats and bring them to the clinic for routine physical exams and vaccinations. He needed some help, so I offered him in-house veterinary care for his cats, and he gladly accepted. I always had a veterinary assistant accompany

me on house calls. They helped find and catch the often reluctant patients, and assisted with examinations, treatments, and any
necessary paperwork. I really appreciated Megan and Heather's
efforts, —— they were good!

House calls to Mr. Konig's residence were always an adventure, and just walking through the front door was a real experience.
His two cats, Blackie and Whitey, took off with blazing speed and
reckless disregard, — as if someone had just yelled out, "AIR
RAID!!" Those two would knock over their food dishes, flip the
water bowls, and send the throw rugs a-flyin in their great escape.
—— They were outta there! We had to clean up the mess before beginning the roundup. Blackie would usually ditch under the bed,
and Whitey opted for safety behind the living room couch. I was
thankful to have some young, fit, and flexible assistants, because
they were the ones who had to get Blackie out from under the bed
in that very cramped bedroom. I'd swear, sometimes they had to
get themselves into positions that resembled a contortionist doing
yoga exercises, but they eventually retrieved the escapee. Now,
Whitey had the whole routine pretty much figured out. Whichever
end of the couch we'd approach, she'd jet out the opposite end
and fly off to another room. This little rodeo went on for awhile,
but in time, we corralled the little buckaroo. Honestly, I think she
thought we were playing a game of hide-n-seek, because when we
finally caught her, she settled down and started purring.

House calls were also interesting in another way. We got to
know the people on a personal level when they shared memorable
photos, experiences, and cherished memories with us. Mr. Konig,
for example, proudly showed us several framed photos of himself
together with familiar showbiz celebrities. He was with comedian
Jack Benny in one photo, and with the famous ventriloquist Edgar
Bergan in another. Mr. Konig nonchalantly reminisced about being on the same stage and billing with those entertainers and many

others. He'd been a professional ventriloquist himself, performing on the East Coast for many years. —— Wow! Who would have known?

Mr. Konig was a very engaging individual. He always insisted upon giving the vet assistants a tip of $15 or $20 before we left. He'd say, "Here, I want you to have this. —— I appreciate you coming to my house, — you're a nice young lady and I know you can use the money." At first they were reluctant to take the cash gratuity, but Mr. Konig was persistent, and eventually they graciously accepted the gift. Without a doubt, ——Mr. Konig was definitely one of a kind.

Paw Prints on the Heart

Ask anyone about their most favorite pet, then sit back and watch what happens next. The person's eyes will light up as they recall and share cherished memories, often with vivid and exacting detail. You'd think that those events just recently happened, but in all actuality, they'd taken place many years earlier. Those indelible memories prove how strong the human-animal bond can be, and why animals are such an integral part of our lives.

Unfortunately, time stands still for no one, and it takes a heavy toll on all of us, including our pets. There will come a time when our faithful companion's health and quality of life has deteriorated to such an extent that we're faced with a difficult and agonizing question and decision, —— "Is it time to relieve the pain and suffering?" The final answer needs to be based upon the love and compassion we have for our devoted friend, —— but that still doesn't make it any easier.

Going on a final house-call always weighed heavily on my heart. I knew it was an act kindness and compassion, yet I could empathize with the people, because I'd been there many times myself. Invariably, the patient was laying on its favorite soft bed, surrounded by family members choking back tears. I'd kneel down and gently stroke the dog's head, —— telling them how good and courageous they'd been, and that I'd come to help them go to a nice place where they wouldn't be sick or in pain anymore. A place where they could run, play, and chase butterflies all day long. The look in their eyes told me that they were ready to go. I then explained to those present that I'd first administer a sedative, and after a few minutes had passed, then the final painless intravenous injection would be given.

The family had come to terms and were at peace with what was necessary for their beloved companion. They wistfully reminisced about the good times, and spoke of how their four-footed family member had enriched their lives and taught them how to forgive and love unconditionally. As I administered the final injection, the family members would gently stroke their companion's head and tell them about a future reunion where they'd all be together again, —— and I truly believe they will be. The "crossing over" was gentle, quick, and painless. Their faithful friend was now at peace. I often gave the family a lock of their friend's hair, and made a keepsake paw print for them. —— Both served as tangible reminders that, although their companion wasn't with them physically any longer, they'd never be forgotten. Then came the tears and the consoling hugs. The families were always very appreciative and thankful for the gentle passage. It was a bittersweet moment, —— an emotional roller coaster. For the family, it was a relief that the struggle was over, but a time of sadness in that their devoted companion was no longer with them. One thing was certain, —— there would forever be paw prints on their hearts.

A Real Downer

A chilles was a Greek hero who fought in the Trojan war, and he was also the main character in Homer's Iliad. The legend tells us that when Achilles was an infant, his mother, Thetis, held him by his heel and dipped him into the river Styx in order to make him invulnerable, but his heel where he was being held remained dry and unprotected. The heel was Achilles's only vulnerable spot on his body, and he was later killed by an arrow wound to his heel. So the term, "Achilles heel" was coined and used as a metaphor for a deadly weakness, that in spite of overall strength, could actually or potentially lead to a devastating downfall.

Not only do we as humans have our own particular areas of vulnerability, or Achilles heel, but so do our animal companions. The Achilles heel of the Dachshund breed seems to be their back. A Dachshund, alias the "wiener dog", has a very interesting body type. It's long and low to the ground because they were originally bred to go down into badger holes and pull the critters out. The problem though, with such a long back, is that the midpoint of the back is particularly prone to intervertebral disk injuries, and when that happens, the consequences can often be devastating. Dachshunds tend to be very active little guys, and with all that gyrating and torquing of their long backs, they can often injure the pliable disks positioned between each vertebrae, causing them to either bulge or rupture, which then puts pressure on the nerves and spinal cord. It results in intense pain, and is often accompanied by temporary or permanent hindquarter paralysis. Immediate medical attention is critical to having any chance of a favorable outcome for such a condition.

"Fritz"

Terry and Chelsea Empler walked through the clinic door carrying their three year old Dachshund, "Fritz", who'd been "down in the hind end" for two weeks. When I heard Mr. Empler make that comment, my heart sunk, because too much time had elapsed since the problem first appeared. — Not a good situation for Fritz.

Little Fritz, bless his heart, did his best to support himself on the exam table. It was difficult to watch him struggle in an effort to make his hindquarters move, but it was all to no avail. He propped himself up with his front legs, held his head up high, and you could tell by the look in his bright little brown eyes that he really didn't understand what was going on. What really got to me was when I stroked his head, — he actually licked my hand, as if he were consoling me instead of visa versa.

My initial exam revealed that Fritz had a major posterior paralysis that involved both hind legs. Neither hind leg responded to the interdigital pinch reflex test. There was absolutely no feeling whatsoever. His tail was totally limp, and he didn't have any bladder control either. X-rays showed a profound narrowing of the intervertebral space between T13 and L1, suggesting that the intervertebral disk had been severely compressed, which caused it to bulge, and rupture. That produced intense pressure on the spinal cord, which in turn resulted in the total restriction of nerve impulses to Fritz's hindquarters, — causing the paralysis.

The treatment options for intervertebral disk syndrome cases included surgical decompression, anti-inflammatory medication plus muscle relaxants, strict inactivity, and acupuncture therapy. The success of the treatment regimens depended upon early initiation and the degree of severity of the injury. Unfortunately for

Fritz, he'd been dealt a bad hand, and his paralysis, at this point, appeared to be untreatable and permanent.

Mr. and Mrs. Empler were crestfallen when I explained to them the extent of Fritz's condition, and the unfavorable prospects for his future. Then it hit me, — "There is one other possibility," I said. "and that's a wheeled cart for paralyzed dogs. You know, — kind of a wheelchair. — I've got one here in the clinic, and I think it could be adjusted to fit little Fritz. Would you be willing to give it a try?" "Oh yes, — yes!" Mr. and Mrs. Empler said in unison as their tear-filled eyes lit up with hope. I told them that it often takes some dogs a little while to adjust to moving about in a wheeled cart, so I cautioned them to be patient with Fritz.

I retrieved the wheeled cart, made a few minor adjustments so it would fit Fritz's body, and then placed the little guy into his "new wheels". He had a great attitude! He was excited, and didn't appear intimidated whatsoever by the strange aluminum contraption. In fact, he looked quite confident as he stood there, supporting himself with his front legs while his hind legs were suspended in padded stirrups positioned over the wheels. We had a long central hallway in the clinic, and it was the perfect place for Fritz to make his "trial run". Mr. Empler got down on his hands and knees at the far end of the hallway and called out, "Fritz, — come!" Fritz raised his head and perked his ears, — then suddenly, — off he went, — full tilt, with ears flapping wildly and wheels a-turnin. It was a sight to see! Fritz was having fun again! Then Mrs. Empler called him, and back down the hallway he went. Little Fritz was really getting the hang of it. Everyone was cheering him on, and the little guy gladly obliged,— showing off his new motor skills. Sometimes he'd get a bit carried away and turn too sharply. When that happened, the cart tipped over, — but no big deal. Fritz just waited there patiently until someone put him back upright, — then off he'd go, — full speed. He was one happy camper! He sort of reminded me of what Alfred E. Newman of Mad Magazine would always say, "What? Me worry?"

Fritz's story is heartwarming and inspiring. He showed everyone what a positive attitude and sheer determination can accomplish. Fritz went on to enjoy a very good, free-wheeling life, and demonstrated to all what it takes to be an overcomer.

Alternatives

Doxie back problems ranged from mild to severe, and the treatment approaches varied accordingly. Most mild cases could be successfully managed, but a full blown posterior paralysis was a whole different story. A hind quarter paralysis of any degree seemed to be the "last straw" for many doxies and their owners. Although the owners dearly loved their dogs, there were instances where the needed back surgery was financially impossible, and the people thought that humane euthanasia was their only option. I didn't want to go down that road, — there had to be other ways to go. Then there was the Dachshund (doxie) Rescue organization. Those folks came to the aid of numerous "downer" doxies, hoping to provide some measure of relief and ultimately find new homes for those compromised little wiener dogs. Scenarios like these prompted me to find, offer, or suggest alternative forms of treatment which could be effective and, most importantly, affordable.

My standard approach, other than surgery, was to use oral anti-inflammatory medication in combination with muscle relaxants and a special medicinal preparation that I'd formulate. It consisted of a penetrating reagent along with a potent steroid. I'd shave and clean an area along the dog's back that corresponded to the problem site, and then apply the liquid preparation topically with the aid of a dauber. The reagent carried the steroid deep into the tissue, reduced the swelling of the bulging disk, and took pressure off the spinal cord. The only problem, — it smelled awful, — but it worked, — and the price was right! There were also occasions when I recommended acupuncture therapy, and the results were often amazingly successful at relieving a paralysis.

What was truly gratifying was the fact that the alternative procedures offered people hope for their beloved friend when initially all seemed lost. That hope was eventually realized in many cases, — and as the word spread, I was called upon from far and wide to come to the aid of the little "downers".

Summer Troublemakers

Everyone enjoys the gentle warm breezes of summer, but those mild winds can sure dry things out. The lawns get dry and turn brown, and so does just about everything else. When that happens, the weed and grass seeds also become dry and are easily scattered. Certain seeds can cause a myriad of problems, and the cheatgrass seed/awn, also referred to as a foxtail, seemed to be one of the worst culprits.

"Billy Bob"

Norm Southwick had a three year old German Shorthair dog named, "Billy Bob", and that dog was one heck of a hunter. Billy Bob lived to hunt and Norm put him through intense summer field training in preparation for the Fall hunting season.

Norm had noticed that Billy Bob was squinting his left eye and rubbing it for several days, so he made an appointment to have it checked out. Billy Bob came through the clinic door with his left eye completely closed and tears were running down the left side of his face. He was definitely experiencing discomfort in that eye, so I immediately placed an anesthetic onto the eye in an attempt to relieve some of the pain. Once the eye didn't hurt anymore, he opened his eyelids, and that made the examination much easier. It didn't take long to find the end of a cheatgrass awn/seed hiding under the eyeball. All Billy Bob's attempts to dislodge the awn hadn't worked because the tiny little barbs on the wispy tail of the awn were holding it in place, and the abundant flow of tears didn't seem to help dislodge it either. I delicately grasped the tail of the awn with a small forceps and gently removed it from its hiding place. Next, I examined the eyeball itself. The cornea, normally clear and transparent, appeared opaque and cloudy, due to the swelling and edema that resulted from the irritation of the cheatgrass awn plus all the self trauma from Billy Bob's rubbing. I applied a fluorescing stain to the surface of the cornea, and it revealed several abrasions plus a small corneal ulcer, both of which would heal with topical medication. Billy Bob's eye problems were solved, and he was now free of the pain and discomfort. He was good-to-go, — hopefully not out into those weeds again.

"Ruger"

Ruger was a sturdy five year old Springer Spaniel who absolutely loved country life. He roamed freely and chased all kinds of birds to his heart's content, but his "no holds barred" lumbering technique didn't work in his favor. He really didn't care what he had to run through, — brush, — weeds, — ponds, — he was just having the time of his life, but that "c'est la vie" attitude is what got him into trouble. Brad Welcher, Ruger's owner, had noticed Ruger licking his paws more than usual the last few days, and thought that Ruger might have allergies or possibly had stepped into something sticky like pine pitch. When the licking and chewing didn't ease up, Brad decided to have Ruger "looked at".

Ruger wasn't limping when he walked into the clinic, but I noticed the hair on all four paws appeared wet, stiff, and matted. Closer inspection revealed that all of his paws were swollen, reddened and infected. The wet, matted hair was not only from saliva, but also from the tacky, serous discharge that was coming from the numerous open sores between his toes. This guy had some major issues going on and needed medical attention, — NOW!

I placed Ruger under a general anesthetic, and proceeded to shave the serum soaked hair off all four paws, exposing the full extent of his problems. There were multiple penetration openings in the web area between each toe on all four paws, and serum was visibly draining from each opening. Cheatgrass awns were everywhere, — in the hair, some partially embedded into the skin, and others had totally perforated the skin and were now migrating deep into his tissue. There were also numerous festering, septic, fistulous tracts, — it was a bad scene! Ruger's body was essentially attempting to reject the embedded offenders, but without much success. Some of the tails of the cheatgrass awns were visible in the openings, so I inserted a small forceps into each hole, grasped the awn, and gently removed it from its hiding place. That procedure was repeated over twenty times. Each tract was then flushed with antiseptics and antibiotics, the paws were bandaged, and for the time being, — the ordeal was over.

When I showed Mr. Welcher the handful of cheatgrass awns that were removed from Ruger's paws, he said, "Holy cow! No wonder he was licking his paws so much. — I guess I'd better check his feet more often." I definitely agreed, and also recommended that the paws be kept shaved, especially during the warm months of summer.

Ruger was a good patient. — He healed quickly, — and it wasn't long before he was back out there running around like crazy. Brad Welcher had also learned a very valuable lesson, — in the future, he kept the hair on Ruger's paws neatly trimmed and inspected the paws daily. The results, — no more embedded cheatgrass awns, — and that made everyone happy!

The Body Invaders

It often seemed as if there wasn't a single place on the dog's body that was off limits to cheatgrass awns. Those pesky little varmints appeared to have a mind of their own, and just when you thought that you'd identified their favorite spots to invade, then they'd throw you a curve and show up somewhere else.

A typical case often seen during the summer months involved a dog shaking its head, scratching and rubbing at one or both ears, and carrying its head cocked to one side. It sort of looked like someone trying to shake water out of his ears after going swimming. However, with the dog, all that head shaking was suggestive of two very plausible scenarios. — 1) A serious ear infection, or 2) A cheatgrass awn that had worked its way deep down inside the ear canal. In many cases it turned out to be the latter, and a quick look in the ear with an otoscope proved that to be true. The tiny barbs on the tail of the cheatgrass awn prevented it from being easily removed. So the only way to get it out safely was to sedate the dog, and physically grasp the awn with a specialized forceps called an Alligator Forceps, and pull the sucker out. Sometimes the pointed tip of the awn would contact and even puncture the eardrum, and needless to say, when that happened it was very painful to the dog and serious damage to the eardrum and inner ear infections often resulted. Once the little invader was removed, the dog felt much better, as could be expected, and he was good-to-go. The odds, however, favored him to be a repeat offender somewhere down the road.

A twelve week old Brittany Spaniel puppy came into the clinic with a large, soft domed swelling on the top of its head. A needle tap revealed it to be an abscess, and it was a bad one too. The little tyke was sedated, the abscess was lanced, drained, flushed, and then treated with antibiotics. Amongst the purulent drainage floated the culprit, — a cheatgrass awn. The owner had been using some cheap, "bargain" straw for bedding, and she confessed that she'd seen a lot of cheatgrass in the straw. One of the awns, along with some bacteria, had penetrated the puppy's skin on its head, and caused the abscess. The moral to the story, — don't use dirty straw for bedding material! Oh yeah, the puppy recovered nicely, and the owner got rid of the straw, and replaced it with a soft new bed. — Problem solved!

"Red" was a beautiful Irish Setter who was brought to the clinic with a grapefruit sized lump on his left side. The hair over the lump appeared moist because the dog had been licking at the site for several days. Shaving the wet stiff hair revealed a very unusual looking lesion. There were oodles of small penetrating holes, fistulous tracts, all over the surface of the lump, and tails of cheatgrass awns could be seen partially embedded in many of the holes. When I placed my hands around the lump and applied gentle pressure, multiple cheatgrass awns came popping out of the holes. The owner happened to be standing right next to Red and witnessed the bizarre scene first hand. She wrinkled up her nose and chimed out, "Eeeeeeeooooo! — That's REALLY gross! — That's disgusting! — How could that happen?" I told her that Red probably laid down on a clump of cheatgrass and the awns worked their way into and through the skin. Red's body was just trying to get rid of those pesky little foreign invaders. The owner responded, "Oh, — I think I know how it happened. Red likes to go and lay on the hay bales in the barn, and that's probably where it all started." That sounded plausible to me. I then sedated Red, removed scads of cheatgrass awns, cleaned and flushed the fistulous tracts, placed him on antibiotic medication, and sent him on his way, — hoping that he'd stay out of the barn, — or that the owners would buy better quality hay.

Over the years, I swear that I'd removed cheatgrass awns from just about every surface and orifice that a dog had, — including the nose, mouth, and all the other very sensitive areas too, — if you know what I mean. That benign looking little plant, gently swaying in the warm summer breeze, appeared so innocent and totally incapable of causing any problems at all, — but it did. It was undeniably one of the worst summertime troublemakers.

Down for the Count

W ho doesn't love animals? They're cute and cuddly when young, and become devoted and loving companions as time goes by. We often form strong bonds with them, and they become an integral part of our life. That close connection frequently inspires people to learn more about their animal's health, behavior patterns, and basic principles of veterinary medicine. There were many occasions when interested individuals requested permission to observe procedures at the veterinary clinic. I was happy to oblige, but soon discovered that some people were suited for it, and some definitely were not.

College students who were seriously considering the veterinary profession as a vocation, were required to spend a specific number of hours with a veterinarian, observing examinations, treatment procedures, and surgeries. This was a requirement before ever applying to the college of veterinary medicine. It served as an opportunity for those individuals to test and evaluate their resolve and intestinal fortitude. Some students had never observed a surgical procedure before, and it proved to be a major eye-opener for them, — in more ways than one.

I always set down ground rules prior to anyone observing surgeries. First and foremost, surgical masks had to be worn, and secondly, their hands had to be kept away from my surgical field. Meaning that there was no finger pointing or touching any of the structures. Thirdly, if they suddenly felt overly warm, sweaty, or dizzy, then they were to — PLEASE TELL SOMEONE! Most observers were interested, focused, and did just fine, however, there were others who didn't do as well. Comments like, "Boy, — it's sure warm in here under those surgery lights", or "I feel a little dizzy", or "I don't feel so good", prompted me to immediately tell them to, "sit down on the floor, — lean your back up against the wall, — and take some deep breaths." Sandy, our office manager, was also a trained and licensed human nurse by profession, and when she heard my comments, — she'd come rushing into the surgery room with smelling salts and cold packs in hand. She immediately went into action, — broke open the smelling salts, — placed the capsule under the victim's nose, and said with con-viction, "Take a deep breath!". That first whiff was a doozie!!! I swear, that stuff could just about raise the dead. She then placed cold packs on their forehead and on the back of their neck, and it didn't take long before the person was back from their foggy experience. The students always felt embarrassed, but I reassured them that it wasn't a big deal, and told them that they'd get used to it, —and they did. In fact, many eventually became excellent veterinarians, however for some, — they discovered that veteri-nary medicine wasn't their cup of tea.

I recall one particular case involving a large Bassett Hound that had been kicked in the muzzle by a horse. According to the owner, the dog's right upper canine tooth had been dislodged, and now all that remained was a big, empty, bloody socket. The dog was brought to the clinic, anesthetized, and preparations were made to close the opening. I had a prospective veterinary student observing that day, and she was anxious to watch the procedure. As I began my preliminary exam of the "empty" socket, I noticed the very tip of the canine tooth, — barely visible, — way up in-side the socket. The tooth hadn't been dislodged, — it had been pushed back up deep within the facial bone. I nonchalantly said to the student, "Want to see me make his tooth reappear?" She looked at me with a puzzled expression on her face, and I then told her, "Watch this!" I delicately grasped the tip of the hidden tooth with a forceps and slowly pulled the huge, two inch long canine tooth from its recesses. "See!" I proudly said as I held up my prize. I looked up just in the nick of time to see her eyelids flutter, then she slowly sank into the sunset. — OUT COLD! A call for help immediately went out for Sandy, and once again she came to the rescue.

One thing was for certain. — If we were going to allow clients and students to observe procedures, then we'd better keep the clinic well stocked with smelling salts and cold packs. Sandy had also become accustomed to the frantic call, — "Help! — We've got another down and outer."

Points of Contention

Porcupines, also known as "quill pigs", have a top ground speed that's a little faster than a tortoise on steroids. Those gentle creatures with the wild hairdos walk around making mumbly, whiney, grunting sounds, and prefer to be left alone. They don't attack anything, but when confronted, defend themselves very effectively with their barbed quills. The quills detach when touched, and are not thrown, as many people believe. Once the quill penetrates the skin, the overlapping scales/barbs help move the quill inward, and many become deeply embedded. Quill cases were always considered an emergency because of the intense pain and disabling effects the quills had on the very unlucky dog. Some dogs had only a few quills in their paws or muzzle, while others had upwards of a hundred or so of the barbed needles embedded all over their bodies. The treatment consisted of placing the dog under a general anesthetic, and manually pulling out the quills individually, — a one-at-a-time procedure. It often turned out to be a very long and arduous task.

The victimized dogs responded quite differently to their piercing ordeal. It all depended upon the number of quills and their locations. If the quills had found their mark in the dog's muzzle, mouth or tongue, the dog usually pawed frantically at its face in an attempt to dislodge the mini-spears. Sometimes the dogs would stand almost motionless, because any movement on their part would cause the quills to slightly move, and that produced more pain and discomfort. Pain in itself can be, and often is, a very powerful motivator, — one way or the other.

Trevor Masters brought his dog, "Sparky", into the clinic with its head completely covered with porcupine quills. Sparky's face was almost unrecognizable, and it actually looked like there was a huge hedgehog sitting atop of his neck. Sparky was an eighty pound Lab-Shepherd mix, and the evidence suggested that he'd gone in for the kill, but came out the loser. He'd definitely got his comeuppance.

Sparky was anesthetized, and three of us, myself and two veterinary assistants, began the challenging task of removing all those quills. Poor Sparky had quills everywhere throughout his mouth, lips, nose, cheeks, ears, and even some had impaled his tongue through and through. There were also a large number of porcupine quills in his front paws and chest. He looked like a totally defeated gladiator! It took the three of us well over an hour to remove all those quills, including multiple "cut-downs" where the embedded quills had to be surgically removed. One of the last places to check were the eyes. When I lifted the eyelid of Sparky's left eye, I saw the very end of a quill protruding from the conjunctival tissue which is located next to and around the eyeball. I grasped the tip and began slowly pulling it out. That quill turned out to be 2 1/2 inches long, and it had assumed a curved shape because when it became embedded, it conformed to the shape of the bony orbit of the eye socket. That was really weird! Sparky recovered nicely, and as he was walking out of the clinic, I said to Trevor, "I sure hope that he's learned his lesson."

Over the years I'd found that most dogs who'd been quilled didn't want to repeat that painful experience again, so in the future, they avoided the "Quill Pig" like the plague. However, there were some, and unfortunately Sparky was one of them, who were repeat offenders. They were bound and determined to get even with that critter who caused them so much pain and discomfort. So, I guess the saying applies to both man and beast, — "Some learn,— Some don't!"

Moments in Time

Certain moments in time are like shooting stars in that they can leave us with some lasting impressions and specific mental images. The following are but a few of the interesting experiences that now reside in my memory bank.

"Carriers"

It was always amusing to see what people came up with for transporting their pets. Its been said that necessity is the mother of invention, and believe me, I saw some pretty interesting improvised carriers. There were the always handy and versatile laundry baskets. All sorts of things were used on top of the baskets to keep the pet inside, and the manner in which those things were attached was quite interesting too. Everything from duct tape to old shoe laces, bungee cords, leather belts, electrical cords, pieces of clothesline, and even old nylon stockings were used. But the most unusual cat carrier that I'd ever seen was a birdcage. Shirley Kohler came waltzing into the clinic one day, toting a birdcage with her cat, "Sam", sitting dispassionately inside. Sam's hair coat and color patterns resembled the cartoon cat named "Sylvester", so I laughingly asked him, "What'd you do with poor little "Tweety Bird"?" He just sat there and gave me a look of quiet resignation, appearing somewhat embarrassed with the whole situation. Shirley quipped, "I was a little behind this morning, — couldn't find the dang carrier, — so I grabbed whatever was handy. — Pretty funny, huh?" I couldn't have agreed more, — but it worked! We both had a good chuckle, however Sam didn't seem to be very impressed.

Other items used as quasi carriers included pillowcases, storage totes, food and beverage coolers, old leather purses and satchels, and of course the good ole reliable cardboard box with air holes punched in it all over the place. There was usually one eye staring out a hole, or a nose poking through another one, or a paw extended out of an opening and swiping aimlessly through the air. — It really did look pretty comical. The unconventional carriers all seemed to do the trick though, — a commercial carrier would have made the job a whole lot easier, — but not quite as entertaining.

"Sam" in his unique carrier

"Pick Pocket"

Puppies and kittens are prime examples of pure energy and joy set into motion. Although playtime seems to be priority number one, they are, without a doubt, constantly learning from their litter mates, surroundings, and us. Those little guys are very impressionable and are quick learners too. So, we need to be mindful of how we interact with them, because bad habits can be inadvertently engrained. — I know, — been there, — done that!

"Scout" was a healthy, bright-eyed, fourteen week old German Shepherd pup and he was a big one "to boot". His calm, confident, self assured demeanor definitely set him apart. Scout was a real charmer, and it wasn't long before the entire staff was drawn to him, oohing and awing over how handsome, well behaved and dignified he was. He just sat there, — cool, calm, and collected, — taking in all the accolades which he'd probably heard a hundred times before. His owner then proudly told me that Scout had come from an exclusive dog kennel in Germany that was known for breeding large, docile, German Shepherds. That little bit of info explained a lot.

As I was in the process of examining Scout, his keen sense of smell honed in on a dog treat located in my uniform pocket. I'd completely forgotten about it being there. Scout unabashedly thrust his long snout deep down into the pocket, and in a flash, proudly withdrew the tasty morsel. We all got a laugh out of his little caper, but then he went back in the pocket for seconds. However, this time the cupboard was bare. Scout was determined to find another goodie in there, and I swear he checked out every thread in that pocket. When he withdrew his nose, he actually looked disappointed, and I couldn't have that, so I stealthily slipped another treat in there and one in the opposite pocket too. Scout dove into my pockets with reckless abandon, — BONANZA! He was

439

in "Hog Heaven". He was having a great time, and it was fun to watch. It didn't dawn on me, at the moment, that I was actually training, i.e. conditioning Scout to check out pockets for treats. Not just my pockets, but everyone else's too. — Not good!

Over the ensuing years, whenever Scout would visit the veterinary clinic, he eagerly trotted into the exam room and the very first thing he'd do was to stick his big, long, wet nose down into my uniform pockets, — looking for the treats, — and he always found some too. Only now, Scout's head and muzzle had become much, much larger, but the pocket size hadn't changed. No problem! He had to do a little extra maneuvering, but eventually he managed to get the tip of his long nose into the pocket, without tearing it off, and retrieved his prize.

Scout remained a big, lovable, happy-go-lucky German Shepherd, who just so happened to have a fetish for checking out people's pockets. I confess. I'd taught him a very bad habit when he was a puppy, — I'd unintentionally trained Scout to be a "Pick Pocket".

"Scout" searching for treats

"Elevator up!"

The profession of veterinary medicine, like many other professions, requires a specific number of continuing education hours periodically in order to maintain one's license to practice medicine. Veterinary conferences provided an excellent opportunity to attend relevant courses and learn new methods of diagnosis and treatment. Those gatherings also offered a chance to checkout all the current reference materials, new pharmaceuticals, and instruments. — Plus, it was an occasion to peruse all the new and interesting equipment that had recently become available. It was like a very big, expensive candy store! As I wandered past all the vendors, something extremely interesting caught my eye — A hydraulic lift examination table! — What a great idea! Now I wouldn't have to break my back attempting to lift a 100+ pound dog onto a stationary exam table. I looked at the price tag, — believe me, —it wasn't cheap, but it was a much better alternative to back surgery. So I took a long, deep breath, — and bit the bullet! My heart was pounding as I made the decision to buy that table, but I knew, without a doubt, that it was a necessary purchase.

The lift table was a wonderful addition to the practice. It truly was a back saver, and most dogs tolerated the table quite well. Oh sure, there were a few like "Bruce", a big 75 pound, tricolor, rough coat collie, who was petrified by the lift table. Whenever he got on the table, he'd immediately lay down and tried to disappear. He'd start salivating, and then his teeth began to chatter, — nonstop, — until he got off the table. He was, what we referred to as a "quiet protester", but his teeth weren't all that quiet, in fact, you could almost hear his teeth chattering in the next exam room. Usually one vet assistant would console and reassure Bruce throughout the exam, but it didn't seem to help very much. When the "ordeal" was over and Bruce slithered off the table, he instantly returned

441

to his usual confident self and pranced out through the waiting room with his head held high, acting as if the whole experience never happened. Ole Bruce, — he was a real character, — and you couldn't help but love him.

Then there was "Sebastian", a handsome, black and white, 90 pound Malamute with an energy level that would rival Mick Jagger. When that big boy entered the clinic, it was plain to see that he was a real handful for his owner, Tracy Heath. It took a major effort, on her part, to control all the twisting and dancing on the end of that hefty leash. Sebastian was one exuberant dude though, and he let everybody in the entire county know it by his loud happy yips and long, low pitched — Woo Wooooo's. This guy really loved life! As I watched all the commotion, I thought to myself, "How in the world am I going to examine this noisy, powerful whirling dervish?" There was no doubt about it, — examining him on the floor would be a rodeo and appeared to be nearly impossible. With Tracy's help, we eventually maneuvered Sebastian next to the lift table and with the coordinated efforts of three people we placed the loud, gyrating Sebastian onto the platform.

At the precise moment Sebastian was placed on the lift table, an astounding transformation took place, — he gently laid down and chilled out. WOW! What a change! As I was about to flip the switch to raise the table I told him, "Sebastian, hold on, — the elevators going up". The muffled whine of the hydraulics didn't phase him one iota. Sebastian remained cool, calm, and collected, thank goodness, throughout the entire physical examination, and then I lowered the table so he could easily step off. He hesitated initially, but with a little coaxing, we finally got him off the lift table, and immediately he started vocalizing and jumping around like a wild man again. I tapped the surface of the table with my hand to get his attention, —then asked him, "Do you want to go for another ride?". In the blink of an eye the big guy jumped back onto the lowered table, quietly laid down, and looked directly at me with an expression as if saying, "Whatcha waitin for? — Let's go again!" So, I flipped the toggle switch and said "Elevator up, — first floor, — leashes and treats." He just laid there, — quietly zoning, happy as a clam. I repeated the up and down elevator ride for him several times, and at that point I was beginning to feel like a carnival ride operator.

The exam had been completed, and there were other patients waiting to be seen, but Sebastian was enjoying himself so much that he didn't want to leave. I told Tracy that Sebastian was welcome to come to the vet clinic anytime he wanted, and get his "FREE" ride, — and he did, — more than once. Sebastian was a great dog, and he sure loved to hear the words, —— "ELEVATOR UP".

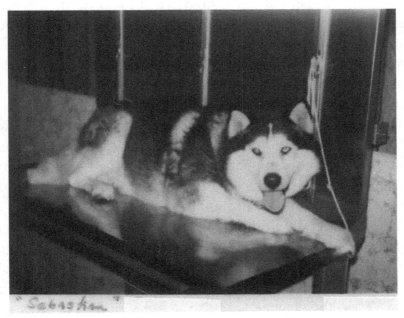

"Sebastian" enjoying his elevator ride

"Stand by me"

It's always heartwarming to watch service dogs in action. They are dedicated canines who unselfishly provide assistance to the special needs of their human companions. These exceptional helpers aren't just limited to aiding people, sometimes they even help each other.

"Keto" and "Tonka" were litter mates, but they sure didn't look like it. Tonka had the body type, color, and personality of an Australian Shepherd, while Keto resembled a small framed Labrador Retriever. Keto also had one other major difference, — she was totally blind, — from birth. She had a congenital anomaly called bilateral microopthalmia, meaning that both eyes were abnormally small, malformed, and nonfunctional. She'd never experienced the miracle of sight, so to her, she was normal. Keto instinctively compensated for her blindness by relying on her other senses of hearing, smell, and touch. That's where Tonka came to the rescue. She was Keto's point of contact and essentially become a "seeing eye dog", — to a dog. Keto would either lightly touch or be in close proximity to Tonka most of the time. Tonka seemed to be acutely aware of her sister's needs, and avoided venturing into areas or situations which could potentially pose a serious threat or problem for either or both of them. Without question, it was Tonka's patience and gentle guidance that allowed Keto to enjoy a relatively normal life.

"Doodles" and "Petunia" were another interesting duo. Petunia, a Pomeranian -Boston Terrier combo, was the matriarch of the household, and Doodles, a black Miniature Poodle, was her protege. Those two got along well, but it was definitely obvious as to who was the teacher, and who was the pupil. That was demonstrated each day as Petunia made her inspection trek around the premises. Petunia always took the lead, while Doodles followed close behind, — learning the routine from the master. As time passed, and the dogs aged, Petunia's eyes gradually changed, and her vision had become quite dim. These changes went unnoticed by their owner until one day she saw that Doodles was leading the walkabout, and Petunia, now virtually blind, followed closely behind. What an astounding role reversal! Doodles had learned her lessons well, and now Petunia, with Doodles help and guidance, was able to enjoy life, in spite of her visual challenges.

I guess the singer/songwriter's lyrics said it all in the cases of Keto and Tonka, — and Petunia and Doodles, —— "I can get by with a little help from my friends".

Petunia & Doodles

A Promise Kept

Carol Francis was an energetic, independent woman who had a sincere passion for animals and their welfare. She'd experienced more than her share of trials and personal tragedy during her life, but she'd always remained positive and strong through it all. Carol often said that it was the devoted companionship and unfailing love of her faithful animals that provided her the solace she needed to get through those very difficult times.

As Carol sashayed through the front door of the clinic and into the waiting room, it was plain to see that she'd mastered the art and technique of carrying two occupied cat carriers and her big purse, — all at the same time. She'd brought two of her cats, "Chrissy" and "Missy" to the vet clinic for routine physical exams, blood work, and vaccinations. Chrissy, a fifteen year old red-point Siamese cross, the matriarch of the household, was in relatively good health for her age, while Missy wasn't as lucky. Missy was a tortoise-shell colored, portly little princess about three years younger than Chrissy. Unfortunately, she'd been battling chronic renal failure (CRF) for several years. The eventual outcome wasn't encouraging, in spite of being fed a kidney friendly diet, receiving appropriate medications for associated conditions, and being give intravenous and subcutaneous fluids on a regular basis. We were all aware that as her kidney's filtering ability decreased, toxins would build up in her system, she'd be essentially poisoning herself, — and regardless of all our heroic efforts, — she wouldn't survive. Our goal was to help her feel as comfortable as possible, for as long as possible, and at the present time, we were ahead of the curve, — she was stable, feeling good, and still enjoying life.

During the course of the physical exam, Carol asked, "Doc, — if something were to happen to me, — what would happen to Chrissy and Missy? Chrissy is old, — and Missy has so many problems, — who would take them? — I wouldn't want to have them put to sleep. — Doc, — what should I do?" I thought for a moment, then said, "Carol, those are some pretty weighty questions you're asking. I'm sure we could find them homes, — but finding the right person might be a challenge though. — Anyway, — nothing's going to happen to you, — so don't worry about that just now." I could tell by Carol's facial expression that she was still very upset. Then she blurted out, "Doc, — could you take them? — I know you'd be able to find them good homes. — Promise me, Doc. — Please PROMISE me that you'd take them and find them homes instead of putting them to sleep." Carol was actually pleading. — She sounded very desperate, — almost panicky. So, to calm her down I said, "Carol, — Okay! — I promise to take them, — but nothing's going to happen! — Alright? — Nothing's going to happen." That was exactly what she wanted to hear, because as soon as I'd uttered those words, — her face instantly lit up, — she smiled, — and then said, "Thanks Doc." — Then she came around to my side of the exam table and gave me a big hug. I told her, "Well Carol, — now that that's settled, — can we finish the exam?" She chuckled, and appeared obviously relieved. — Then said, "Okay, — sorry Doc".

It was Friday morning, four days had passed since Carol's visit, and I was in the first exam room with a patient. The phone rang, — there was a pause, and then I heard our receptionist Darlene say, "Oh, — I'm so very sorry. — Yes, — I'll tell Doc". I surmised that Dar was talking to someone about an animal patient, so I finished up with my case, then asked Dar, "What was that phone call all about?" Dar looked me straight in the eyes and said, "That was Carol Francis's daughter on the phone. — Carol went into a diabetic coma last night, — and never woke up. — Doc, — she died! — Her daughter also wants to know what she should do with the cats." I just stood there momentarily, — dumbstruck by the shocking news. I had a flashback about Carol's recent office visit, and the frantic request she'd made, — and what I'd told her. "Dar," I said, "Call Carol's daughter, — give her my condolences, — and tell her to bring the cats to the clinic. We'll find them good homes. — They won't be put to sleep!" I paused briefly, and attempted to process all that had just happened. Then the thought crossed my mind, "How'd she know? — Could she have had a premonition?"

The cats arrived at the clinic a few days later. Dar and her husband were totally smitten by Chrissy, — "Miss Personality". Chrissy couldn't have found a better home, — and Carol would have been overjoyed. Missy, on the other hand, was liked by everyone, but was not adoptable. No one wanted to be saddled with that much responsibility and expense, especially with a cat having a terminal condition. So, — she became a "clinic kitty", — and a good one she was! Missy stayed at the vet clinic for a little over one year. She was placed on a strict, low protein diet, she got her medications and fluid therapy on a regular schedule, and had her blood chemistry values evaluated monthly. Missy appeared physically well, but the blood values for assessing kidney function were rising, meaning that the kidneys were wearing out, and the toxins were building up more in her little body. When that happens, a distinct ketone odor can also be detected on the patient's breath, — and it really smells bad. Poor Missy was now at the end stage phase of kidney disease. — It was now time for basically hospice care, so Sandy and I decided that Missy could live out the rest of her days with us, — at our home.

I transformed my 14'x16', two-story, heated, super insulated Tuff-shed, often referred to as Doc's "man-cave", into the premier, plush "cat house of Sherman Avenue". It had all kinds of feline amenities, — multiple cushy cat beds, hammocks, toys, window seats, a television with a special "cat video" set on loop play, and a cat door to a secured outside exercise pen. Missy, the charmer, was definitely in her element. She was a real schmoozer, and it wasn't long before she maneuvered herself into the house, and found an available lap. Her sweet countenance and non-confrontational attitude allowed her to be readily accepted by our other three male cats. Missy soon became one of the family. In the past, Missy had never been permitted outdoors, but we allowed her on occasion, to roam free in our large, fenced, cat-friendly yard. She had a chance to be a "real" cat, — if only for a short while. Missy relished laying on a freshly cut lawn, basking in the sun, chasing butterflies, and occasionally stalking birds. Outwardly Missy looked and acted like any other portly princess, but on the inside, — it was a whole different story.

Missy desperately needed her daily subcutaneous fluid therapy and oral medications in order to counter the awful effects of her failing kidneys. Through it all, she never complained, in fact she actually purred throughout her treatment sessions. Missy really did live life to the fullest, — as long as she could. She'd enjoyed ten good months at our home, but then her condition rapidly deteriorated, and in spite of all our efforts, — our sweet little Missy peacefully went home to be with Carol.

As I gently stroked Missy's little head for the very last time, I recalled Carol's requests, — and I could honestly say, —— the promise was kept.

Sandy and portly princess, "Missy"

EPILOGUE

Looking back over the years, I can definitely say, without a doubt, that I had the greatest patients in the world. They were extremely honest and forgiving, and if they experienced any pain or discomfort whatsoever, — they let me know about it immediately! — There was absolutely no beating around the bush. In spite of any discomfort inflicted, they were always quick to forgive, and they showed it by their happy tails and wet kisses. No question about it. — The animals were, in all honesty, some of my closest and dearest friends, — and I really did love them, — and still do. It was a privilege to be entrusted with their care, and an honor to devote my life to the mending of God's creatures. Would I do it all over again? —— Yup! —— IN A HEARTBEAT!

CPSIA information can be obtained
at www.ICGtesting.com
Printed in the USA
LVHW051031180520
655841LV00006B/328